AF882185

PHYSEO

TABLE OF CONTENTS

We would like to extend a special thanks to the following individuals who have spent many hours tutoring, guiding and consulting this work, making Physeo Embryology possible.

Paloma F Cariello, MD, MPH
Assistant Professor
Division of Infectious Diseases
University of Utah School of Medicine
Salt Lake City, UT

Karen Eilbeck, Ph.D.
Professor
Biomedical Informatics
University of Utah

Vicente Planelles, Ph.D.
Professor
Division of Microbiology and Immunology
Department of Pathology
University of Utah School of Medicine
Salt Lake City, UT

Travis Norseth
MD Candidate Class of 2021
University of Utah School of Medicine
Salt Lake City, UT

Carol Foote
MD Candidate Class of 2021
University of Utah School of Medicine
Salt Lake City, UT

Naveen Rathi
MD Candidate Class of 2021
University of Utah School of Medicine
Salt Lake City, UT

IMMUNOLOGY

Section I - Lymphoid Structures

I. Lymphatic System

A. Group of tissues that remove waste, facilitate immunity, and transport lymph

B. Includes primary and secondary lymphoid organs

C. Right lymphatic duct drains the upper right aspect of the body into the junction between the right subclavian and internal jugular vein

D. Thoracic duct drains the rest of the body into the junction between the left subclavian and internal jugular veins

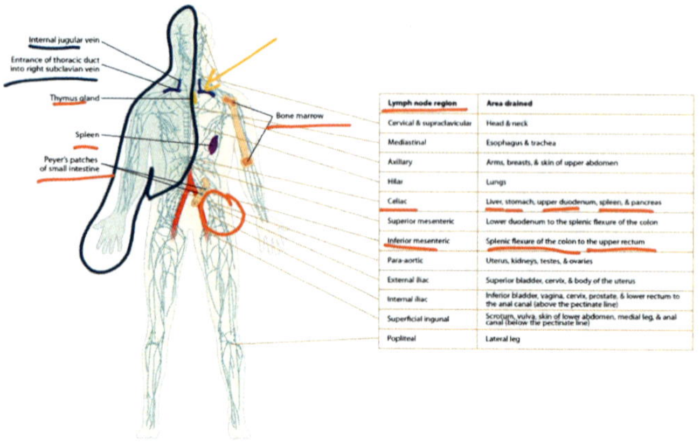

II. Primary vs. Secondary Lymphoid Organs

A. Primary organs:

1. Immune cell production and development
2. Bone marrow (B-cells)
3. Thymus (T-cells)

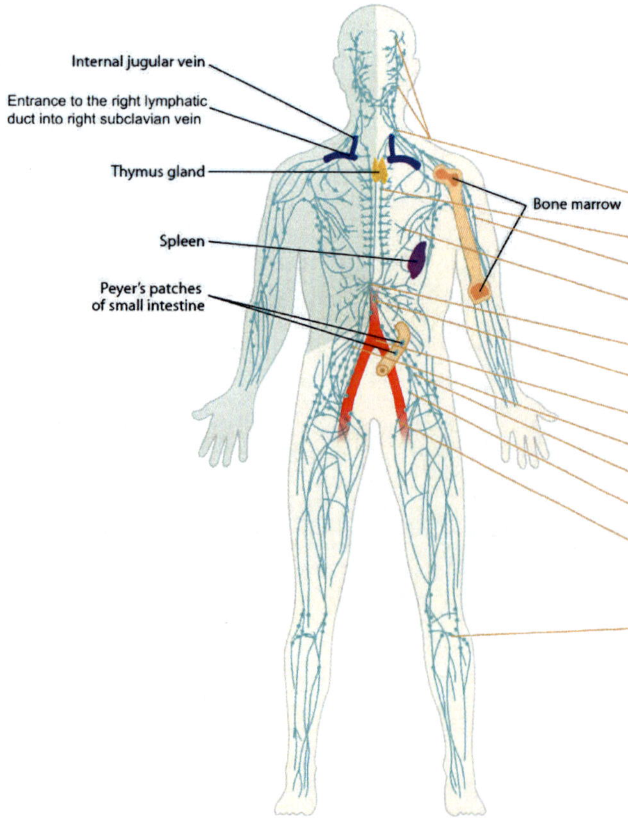

Lymph node region	Area drained
Cervical & supraclavicular	Head & neck
Mediastinal	Esophagus & trachea
Axillary	Arms, breasts, & skin of upper abdomen
Hilar	Lungs
Celiac	Liver, stomach, upper duodenum, spleen, & pancreas
Superior mesenteric	Lower duodenum to the splenic flexure of the colon
Inferior mesenteric	Splenic flexure of the colon to the upper rectum
Para-aortic	Uterus, kidneys, testes, & ovaries
External iliac	Superior bladder, cervix, & body of the uterus
Internal iliac	Inferior bladder, vagina, cervix, prostate, & lower rectum to the anal canal (above the pectinate line)
Superficial inguinal	Scrotum, vulva, skin of lower abdomen, medial leg, & anal canal (below the pectinate line)
Popliteal	Lateral leg

Figure 8.1.1 - The lymphatic system

B. Secondary organs:

1. Antigen interaction
2. Lymph nodes, spleen, tonsils, Peyer's patches

III. Bone Marrow

A. Structure:

1. Red marrow (active)
2. Yellow marrow (fat cells, inactive)

B. Function:

1. Site of B-cell and T-cell production
2. Site of B-cell development

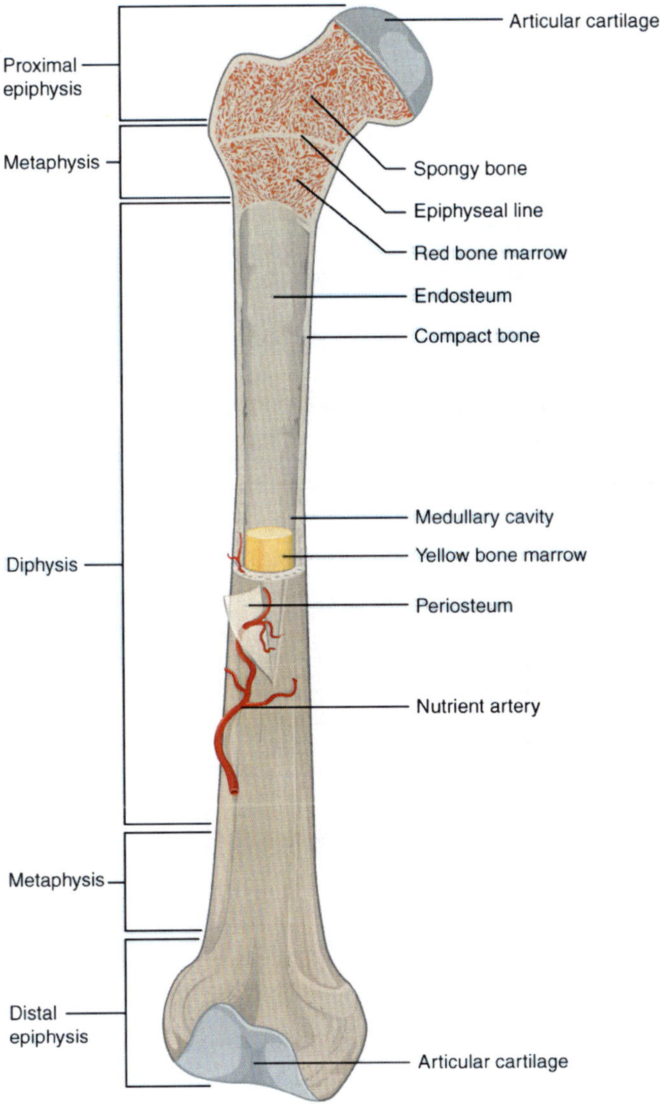

Figure 8.1.2 - Bone anatomy

IV. Thymus

A. Located in the anterior superior mediastinum

1. Derived from ventral wing of the third pharyngeal pouch (endoderm)
2. Thymic lymphocytes are derived from mesoderm

B. Site of T-cell maturation

1. Occurs during the neonatal and pre-adolescent period
2. Atrophies with age
3. Differentiation occurs in secondary lymphoid organs

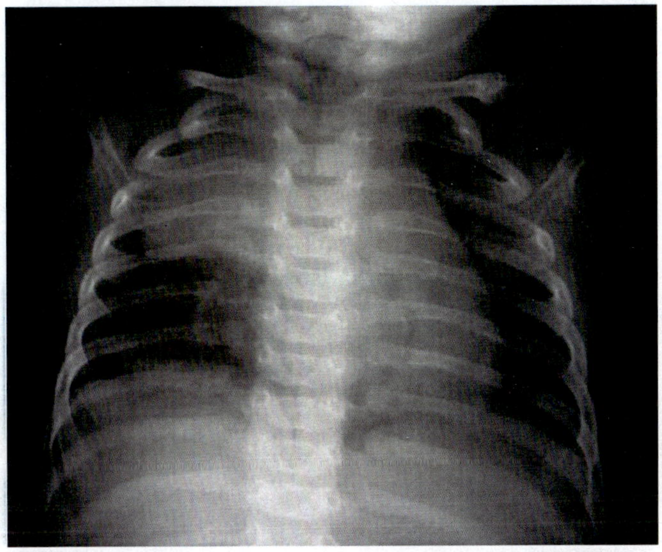

Figure 8.1.3 - Chest x-ray of a neonate revealing the thymus with the characteristic "sail sign"

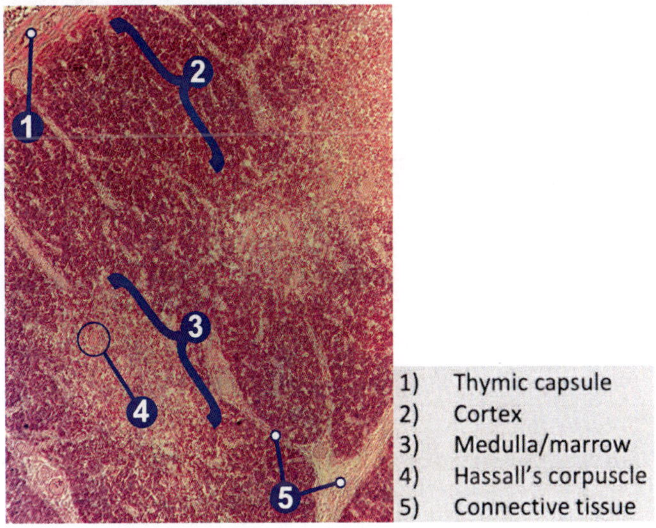

Figure 8.1.4 - Histology of the thymus

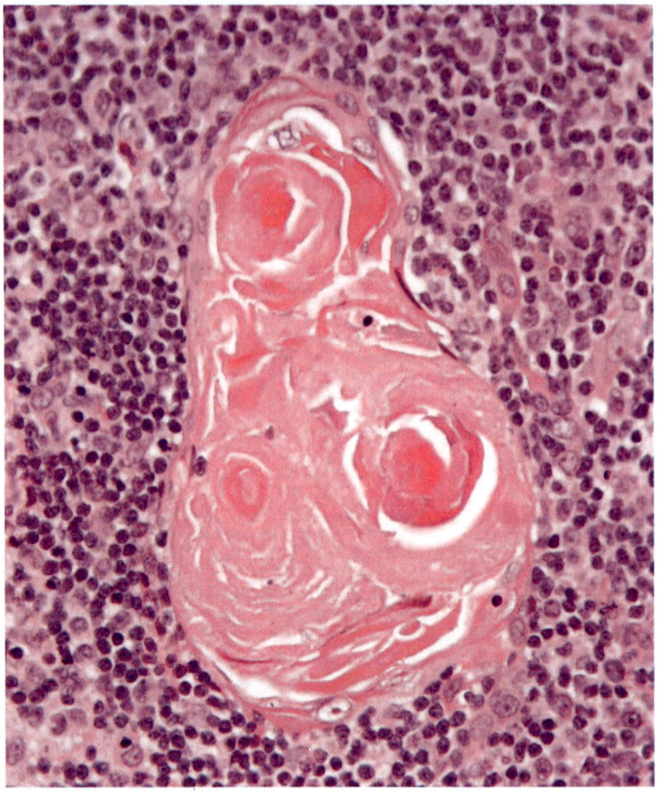

Photo Credit: Nephron [CC BY-SA 3.0 (https://creativecommons.org/licenses/by-sa/3.0)]

Figure 8.1.5 - Hassall's corpuscle

C. Absent thymic shadow:
   1. DiGeorge syndrome and SCID
D. Thymoma
   1. Neoplasm of thymus
   2. Myasthenia gravis, Good syndrome, SVC syndrome, pure red cell aplasia
E. Autoimmune polyendocrine syndrome-1
   1. Loss of thymic AIRE genes → autoreactive lymphocytes

V. Primary vs. Secondary Lymphoid Organs
   A. Primary organs:
      1. Immune cell production and development
      2. Bone marrow (B-cells)
      3. Thymus (T-cells)
   B. Secondary organs:
      1. Antigen interaction
      2. Lymph nodes, spleen, tonsils, Peyer's patches

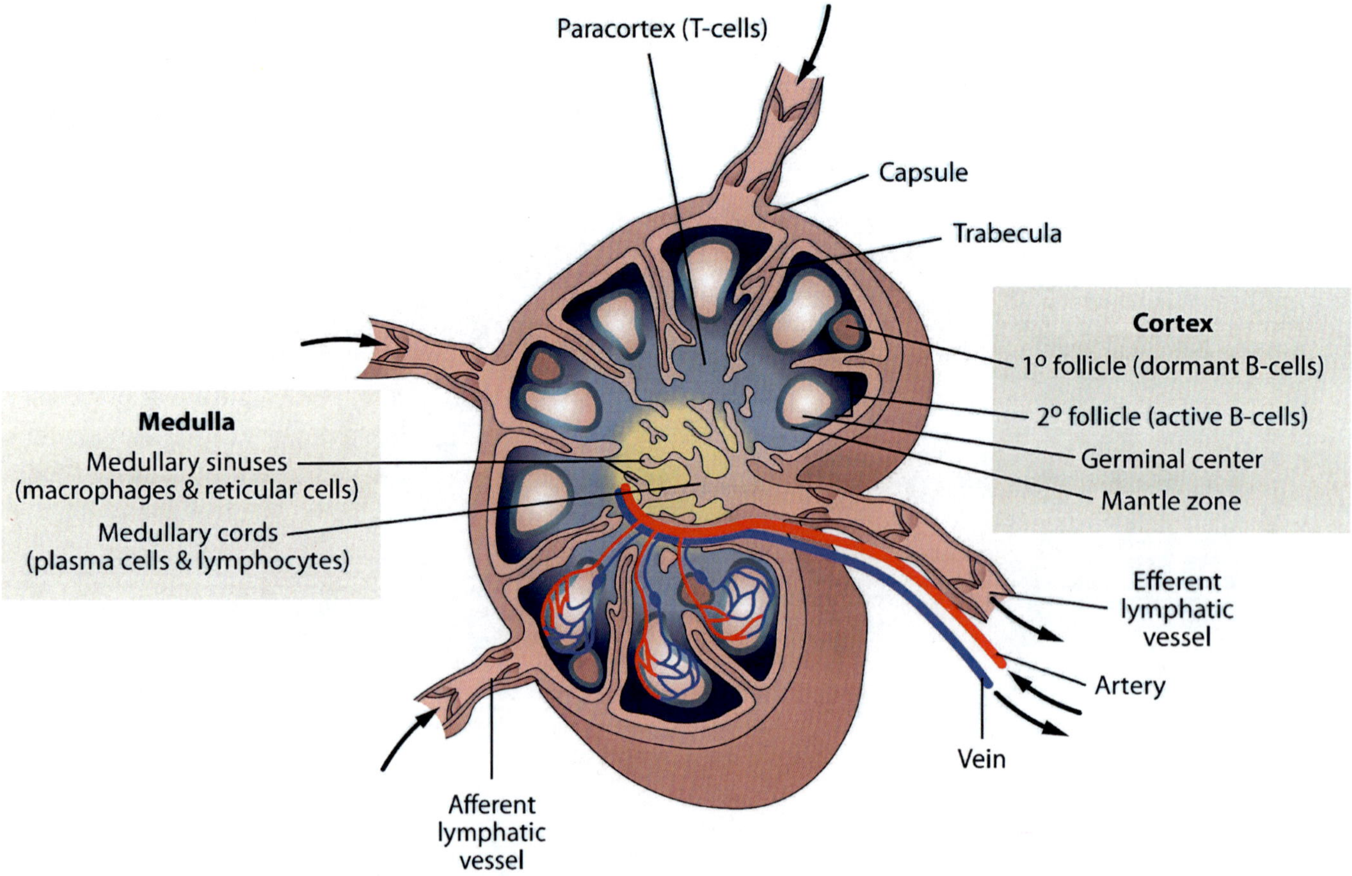

Figure 8.1.6 - Lymph node

VI. Lymph Nodes: Cortex

A. Follicles

1. Site of B-cell localization/proliferation

B. Primary and secondary follicles

1. Primary → dormant
2. Secondary → active

a) Mantle zone and germinal center

VII. Lymph Nodes: Paracortex

A. Consists mostly of T-cells

B. Contains high endothelial venules (HEVs)

C. Disease associations:

1. Underdeveloped in DiGeorge syndrome
2. Region that becomes enlarged in lymphadenopathy

VIII. Lymph Nodes: Medulla

A. Medullary cords

1. Areas of tissue that invaginate into the medulla
2. Contain plasma cells and lymphocytes

B. Medullary sinuses

1. Spaces between the cords
2. Contain macrophages and reticular cells
3. Communicate with efferent lymphatics

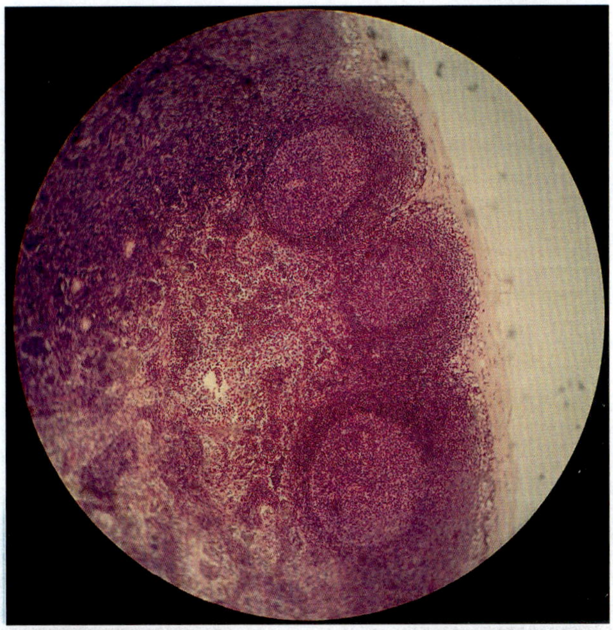

Photo Credit: Lymph node histology by Navid Golpour [Flickr]

Figure 8.1.8 - Lymph node histology

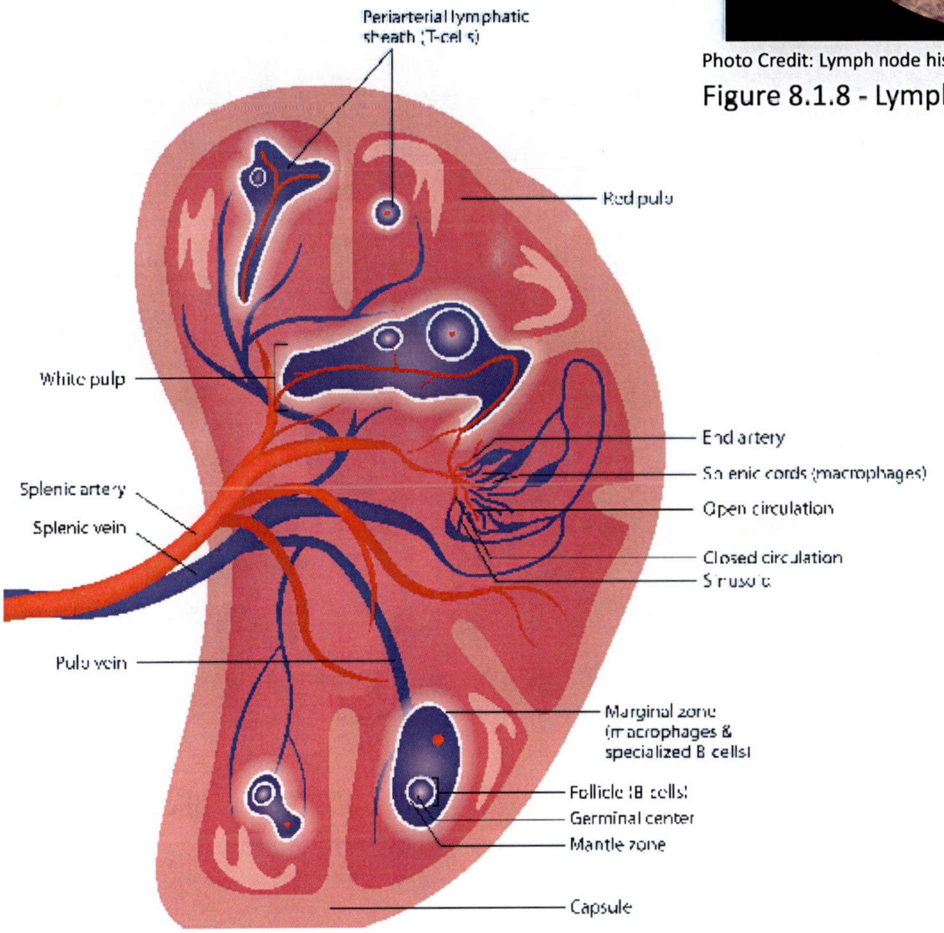

Figure 8.1.7 - Spleen

IX. Spleen: White Pulp

A. Follicle

1. B-cells

B. Periarterial lymphatic sheath (PALS)

1. Dense area of lymphatic tissue surrounding arteries
2. T-cells

C. Marginal zone

1. Area that surrounds the PALS
2. Macrophages, specialized B-cells, and APCs

X. Spleen: Red Pulp

A. Filters the blood

B. Splenic artery → end arteries → splenic cords → sinusoids → venous system

C. Function

1. Remove old or damaged RBCs
2. Serves as another layer of immunity (macrophages interact with antigens and pathogens filtered in the blood)

XI. Spleen: Associations

A. Splenic dysfunction

1. ↓ splenic B-cells → ↓ IgM → ↓ complement & C3b opsonization → ↑ risk of infection by encapsulated bacteria
2. Vaccination against encapsulated organisms is important

B. Postsplenectomy findings

1. Howell-Jolly bodies & target cells (↓ splenic macrophages)
2. Lymphocytosis and thrombocytosis (loss of sequestration)

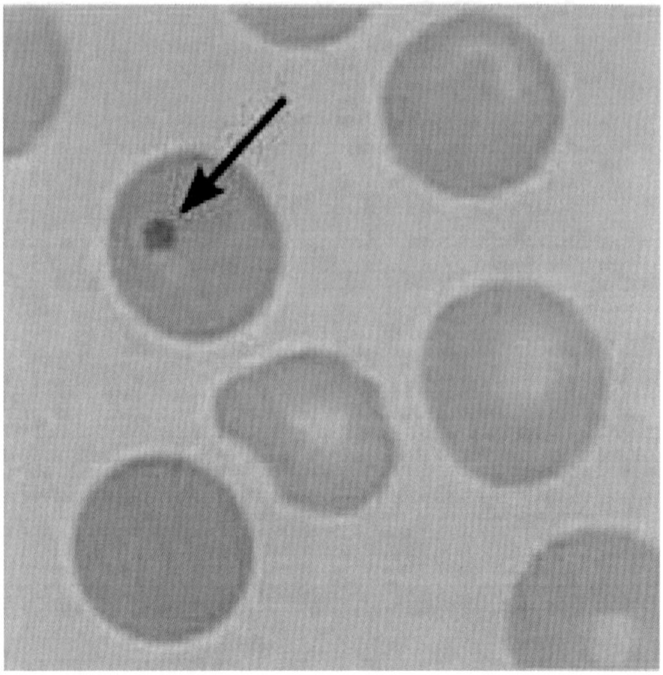

Figure 8.1.9 - Howell-Jolly body

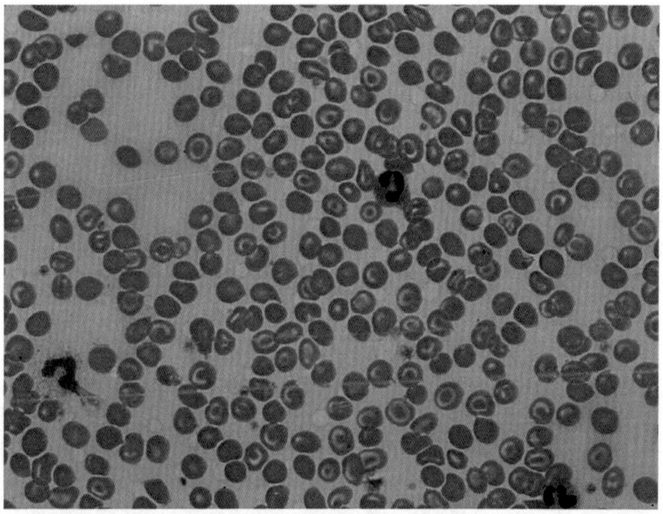

Figure 8.1.10 - Target cells

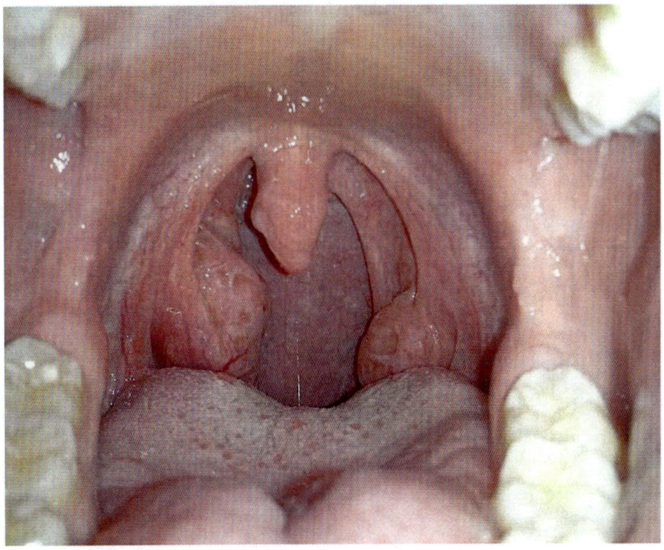

Photo Credit: Valerio Bozzolan [Public domain]

Figure 8.1.11 - Tonsils

XII. Peyer's Patches

A. Lymphoid tissue in the ileum (lamina propria and submucosa)

B. M cells sample and present antigens → B-cell activation

C. B-cells → IgA-secreting plasma cells (found in lamina propria) → IgA is transported to the intraluminal space with protective secretory component

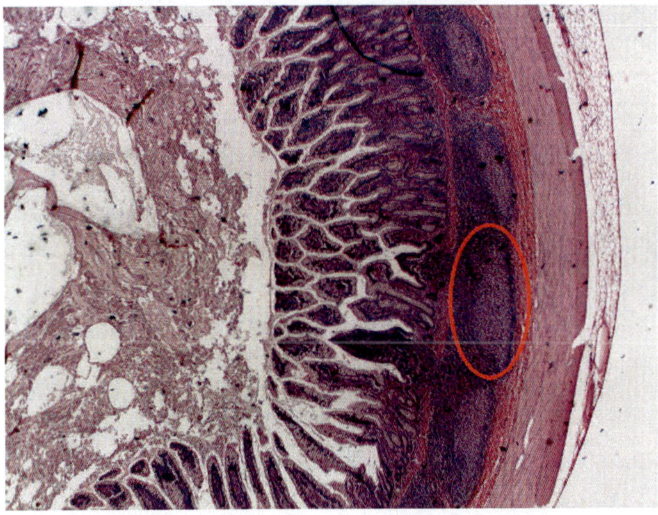

Photo Credit: User:Plainpaper [CC BY-SA 3.0 (https://creativecommons.org/licenses/by-sa/3.0)]

Figure 8.1.12 - Peyer's patch

REVIEW QUESTIONS

1. A 4-year-old boy presents to the physician with a cough, runny nose, conjunctivitis and pharyngitis. His symptoms first started two days ago. Physical examination reveals several tender lymph nodes in the neck. It's concluded that intracellular viral particles are responsible for his symptoms. These infected cells can be neutralized by T-cells which are primarily found in which region of the lymph node?

- **The correct answer is paracortex.**
- **This boy has a viral infection.**
- **He has a cough, runny nose, conjunctivitis, pharyngitis which sounds like a pretty typical cold.**
- **The question also mentions viral particles and states that these infected cells can be neutralized by T-cells.**
- **T-cells are primarily found in the paracortex of the lymph node.**

Section II - Acute Inflammation

I. Acute Inflammation Overview

  A. The immediate and transient response to tissue injury, pathogens, or necrosis

  B. Mediated by the innate immune system

  C. Inflamed tissue will reveal neutrophil infiltration and tissue swelling

II. General Function of Neutrophils

  A. Neutrophils

    1. Rapidly invade connective tissue to phagocytose pathogens or necrotic debris

    2. Phagocytosis depletes neutrophil glycogen → apoptosis → pus

  B. Neutrophil infiltration or pus = acute inflammation

    1. This is true even if inflammation has been going on for several months

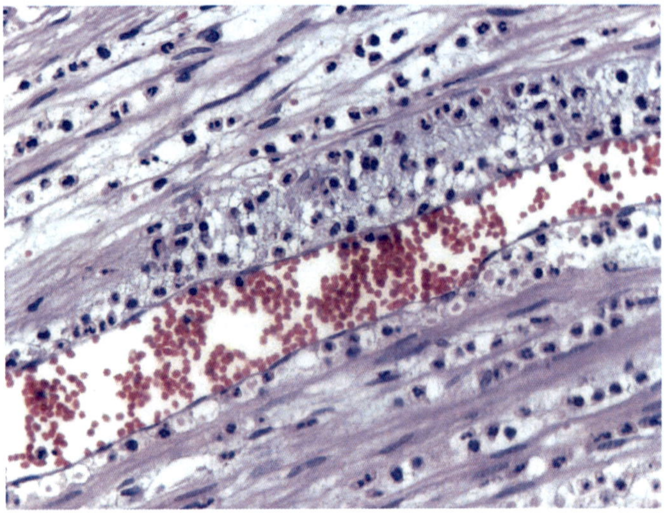

Figure 8.1.14 - Edema and neutrophil infiltration

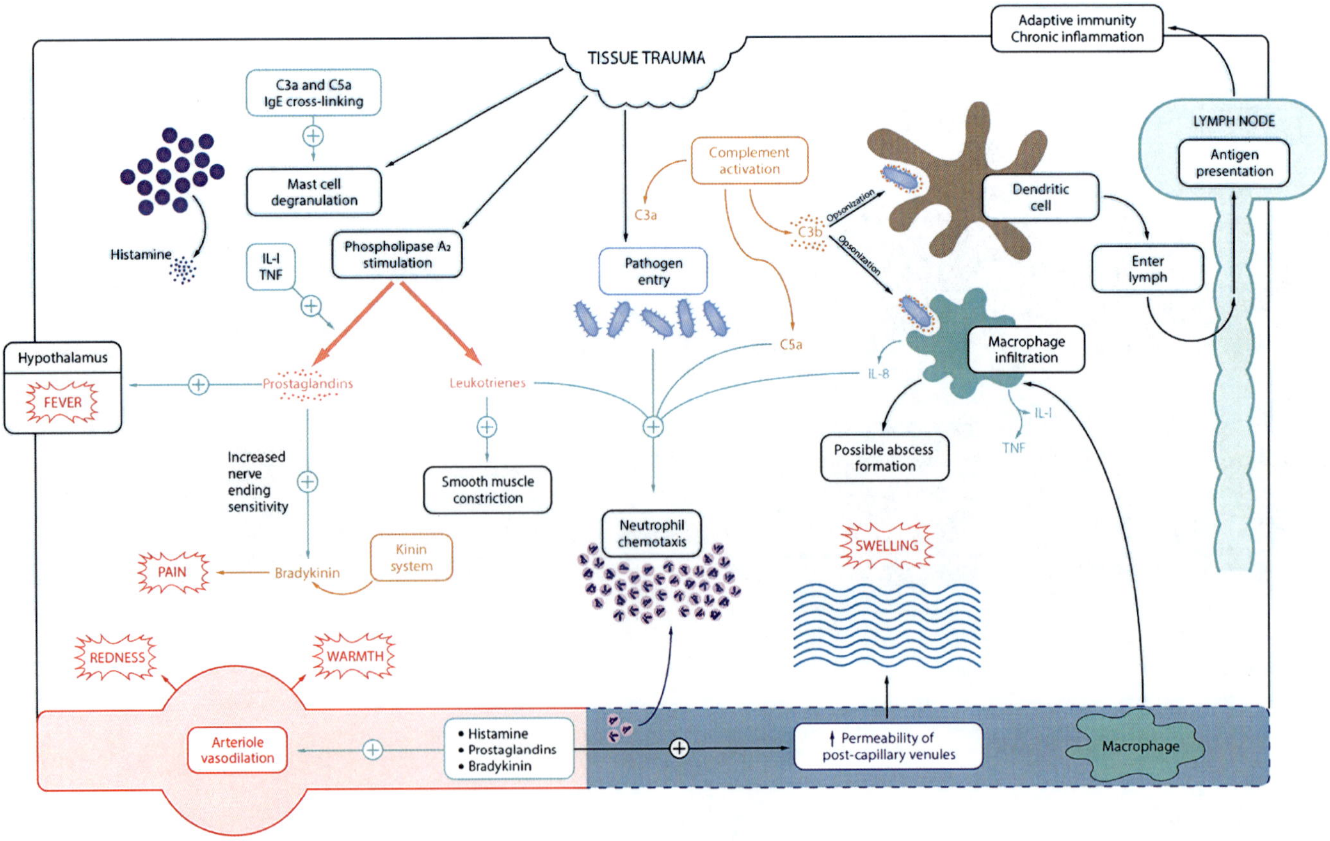

Figure 8.1.13 - Acute inflammation overview

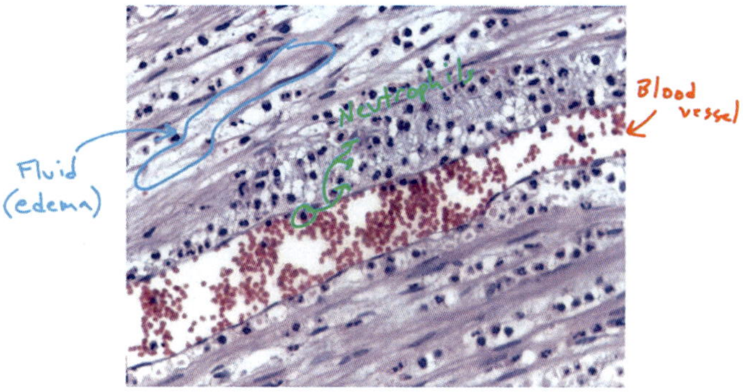

III. Acute Inflammation Timeline

A. Immediately following insult:

1. Mast cell degranulation
2. Phospholipase A_2 (PA_2) stimulation
3. Complement activation

B. 24 hours later:

1. Neutrophil infiltration

C. 2-3 days later:

1. Macrophage infiltration
2. Dendritic cells travel to the lymph nodes

IV. Mast Cells

A. Mast cells are present in nearly all connective tissue

B. Mast cell degranulation releases histamine

C. Triggered by tissue injury, C3a, C5a, or IgE cross-linking

D. Histamine actions:

1. Local vasodilation of arterioles → redness and warmth
2. Local increased permeability of postcapillary venules → swelling

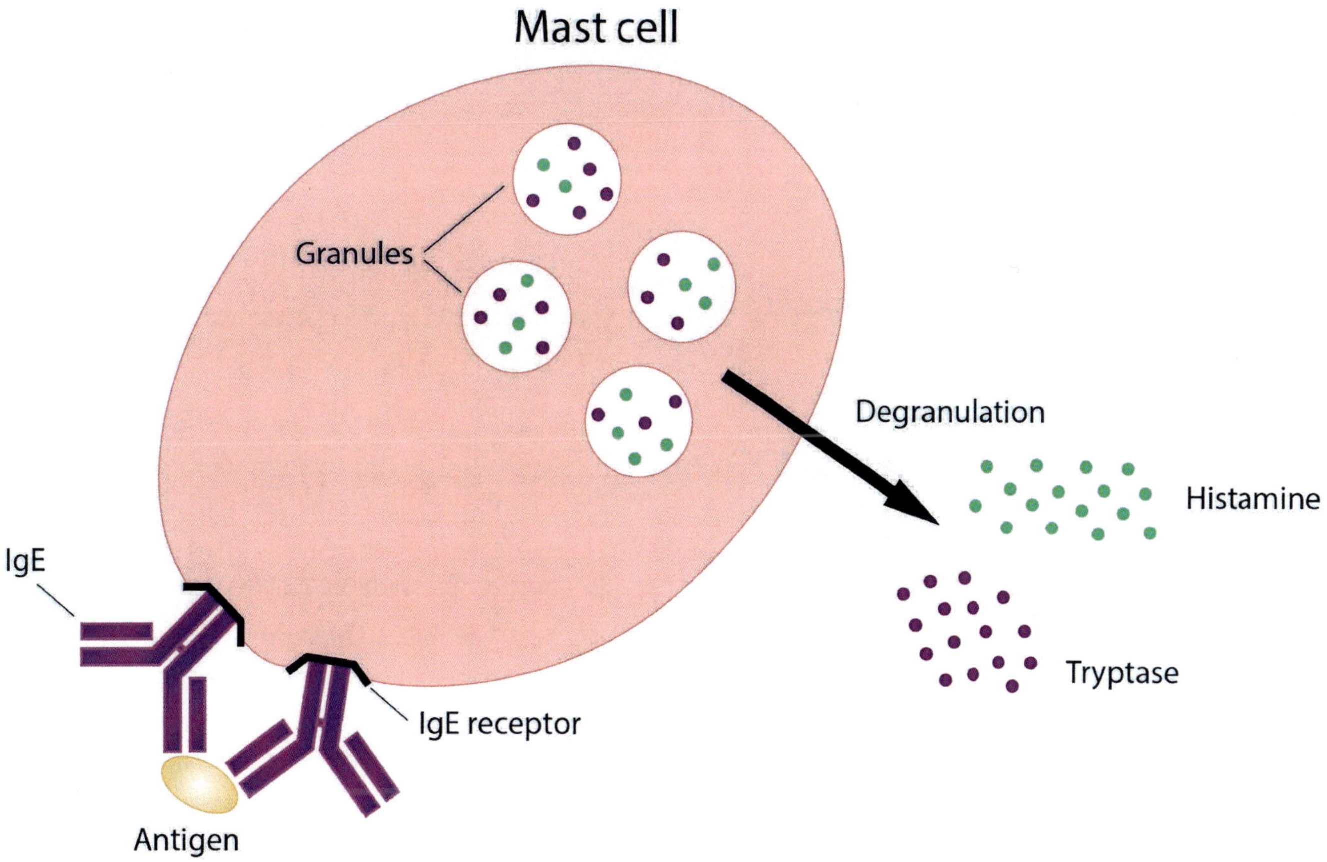

Figure 8.1.15 - Mast cell degranulation and IgE cross-linking

V. Arachidonic Acid Pathway

A. Arachidonic acid (AA) precursors are located on the membranes of many cells

B. Tissue injury stimulates phospholipase A2 (PA2) to release AA from the phospholipid bilayer

C. AA can then be acted on by enzymes:

1. Cyclooxygenase (COX1 or COX2) → prostaglandins

2. 5-lipoxygenase → leukotrienes

VI. Prostaglandins in Acute Inflammation

A. PGI2 PGD2 PGE2 → arteriole vasodilation and ↑ postcapillary venule permeability

B. PGE2 has two important actions:

1. ↑ nerve ending sensitivity to bradykinin → pain

2. Macrophages release IL-1 and TNF → travel to hypothalamus and stimulate cyclooxygenase → PGE2 → ↑ temperature set point in hypothalamus → fever

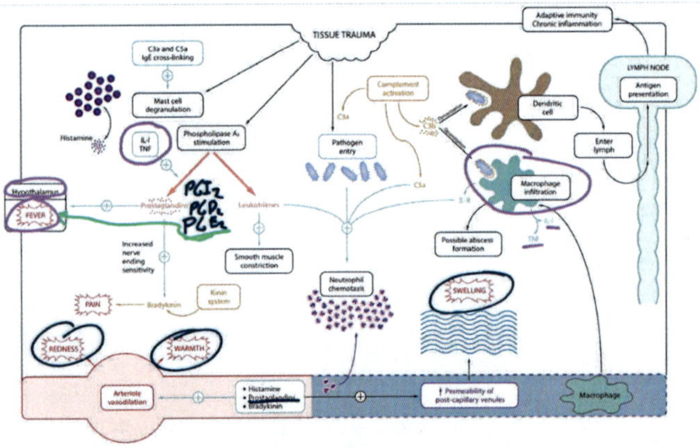

VII. Leukotrienes in Acute Inflammation

A. LTB4 → neutrophil chemotaxis

B. LTC4, LTD4, and LTE4 → smooth muscle constriction → bronchospasm and ↑ vascular permeability (via pericyte contraction)

VIII. Complement in Acute Inflammation

A. Complement activation will increase C5a, C3a, and C3b

1. C5a → neutrophil chemotaxis

2. C5a and C3a stimulate mast cell degranulation

3. C3b → opsonization

IX. Macrophages and Dendritic Cells in Acute Inflammation

A. Dendritic cells and macrophages → IL-8 (neutrophil chemotaxis), IL-1 and TNF (fever, redness, warmth, swelling)

B. Dendritic cells will process antigens → travel to the lymph nodes → present antigens to naive T-cells

C. Possible abscess formation

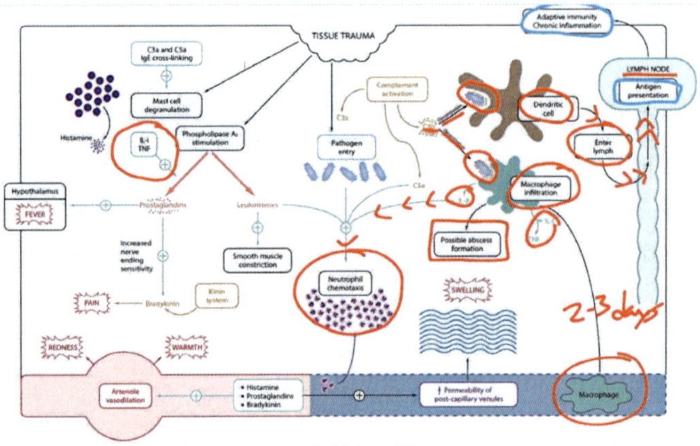

X. Cardinal Signs of Inflammation

A. Redness (histamine, prostaglandins, bradykinin)

B. Warmth (histamine, prostaglandins, bradykinin)

C. Swelling (histamine, prostaglandins, bradykinin)

D. Pain (PGE2 and bradykinin)

E. Fever (PGE2)

F. Loss of function is possible

1. Example: pain may reduce voluntary movement

2. Example: swelling may limit the normal range of motion

REVIEW QUESTIONS

1. How do macrophages contribute to the cardinal signs of inflammation?

- **Correct answer: Through their release of TNF and IL-1**
- **TNF and IL-1 → upregulate COX → prostaglandins → arteriole dilation and swelling → redness, warmth, and swelling**
- **PGE2 specifically causes fever (TNF and IL-1 reach hypothalamus → local PGE2 formation → fever) and pain (increase nerve ending sensitivity to bradykinin)**

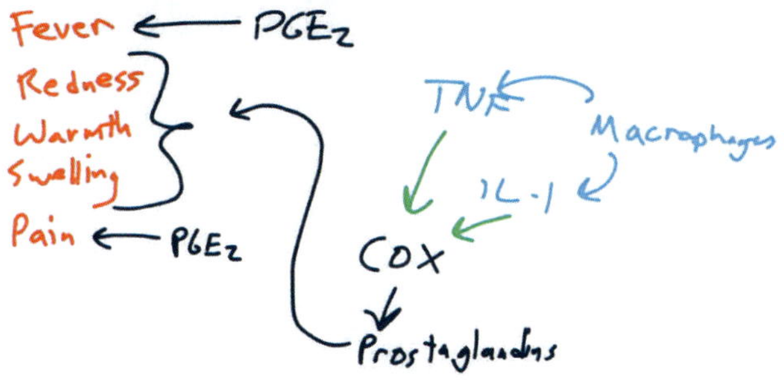

Section III - Neutrophils

I. Important Neutrophil Activities

   A. Extravasation

   B. Phagocytosis

   C. Destroy the pathogen

      1. Oxidative killing (oxidative/respiratory burst)

      2. Non-oxidative killing (lactoferrin)

   D. Apoptosis and pus

Step	Action	Description
1	Margination	- Vasodilation → flow of blood is slowed down → neutrophils flow from center to vascular periphery (margination)
2	Rolling	- Histamine → Weibel-Palade bodies in endothelial cells release P-selectin → P-selectins displayed on vascular wall - TNF and IL-1 → upregulate E-selectins on vascular wall - E-selectins and P-selectins bind weakly to Sialyl Lewis^x on the neutrophils → repeated attachment and detachment between Sialyl Lewis^x and selectins (rolling)
3	Adhesion	- TNF and IL-1 → upregulate cellular adhesion molecules (CAMs) on vascular wall - Notable CAMs include intercellular CAM (ICAM) and vascular CAM (VCAM) - C5a and LTB4 → upregulate integrins called leukocyte function associated antigen 1 (LFA-1, aka CD18) on neutrophils - CAMs bind tightly to CD18 (adhesion)
4	Transmigration	- Platelet-endothelial cell adhesion molecule (PECAM-1, also called CD31) is present on the neutrophils and the endothelial cells - PECAM-to-PECAM attachment → neutrophils enter the interstitial tissue (transmigration)
5	Migration (chemotaxis)	- IL-8, C5a, LTB4 and bacterial products direct neutrophils where in the tissue phagocytosis is required (chemotaxis)

Table 8.1.1 - Neutrophil extravasation

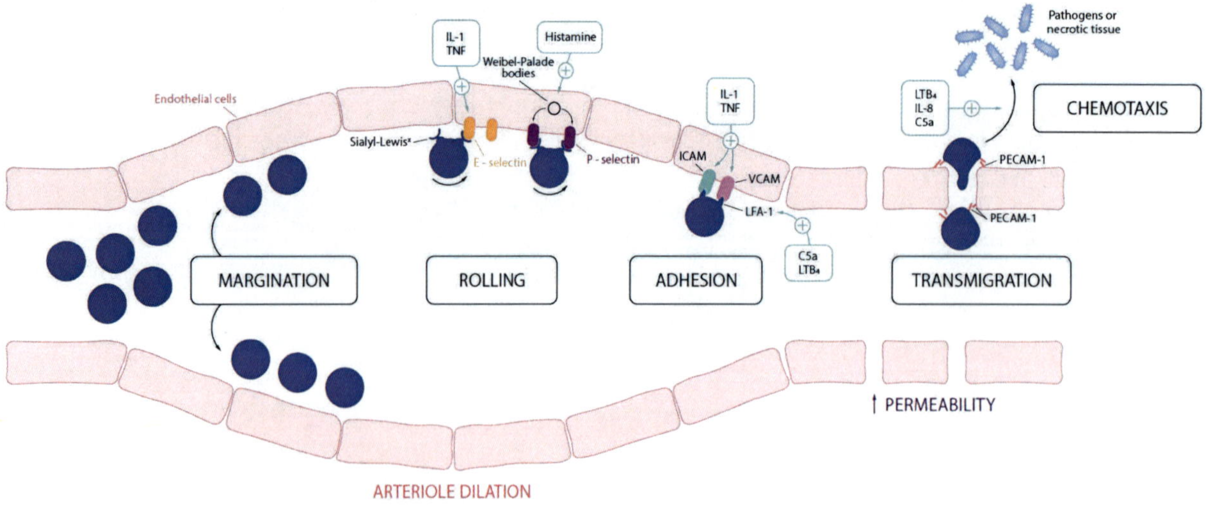

Figure 8.1.16 - Neutrophil extravasation

II. Phagocytosis

A. Neutrophils reach the necrotic tissue or pathogens → necrotic tissue or pathogens are engulfed by the neutrophil which are contained in phagosomes

B. Intracellular phagosomes will combine with lysosomes to form phagolysosomes

C. Within phagolysosomes, pathogens will be destroyed

III. Non-oxidative Killing

A. Less effective than oxidative killing

B. Different immune cells release granules with various substances

1. Neutrophils: lactoferrin (binds free iron → iron is unavailable for pathogen → death)
2. Macrophages: lysozyme (hydrolyzes peptidoglycan → lysis of bacteria)
3. Eosinophils: major basic protein (MBP) is secreted and is toxic to helminths and bacteria → pathogen death

IV. Oxidative (Respiratory) Burst

A. NADPH oxidase converts oxygen (O_2) to superoxide ($O_2^{-\cdot}$)

B. Superoxide dismutase converts $O_2^{-\cdot}$ to hydrogen peroxide (H_2O_2)

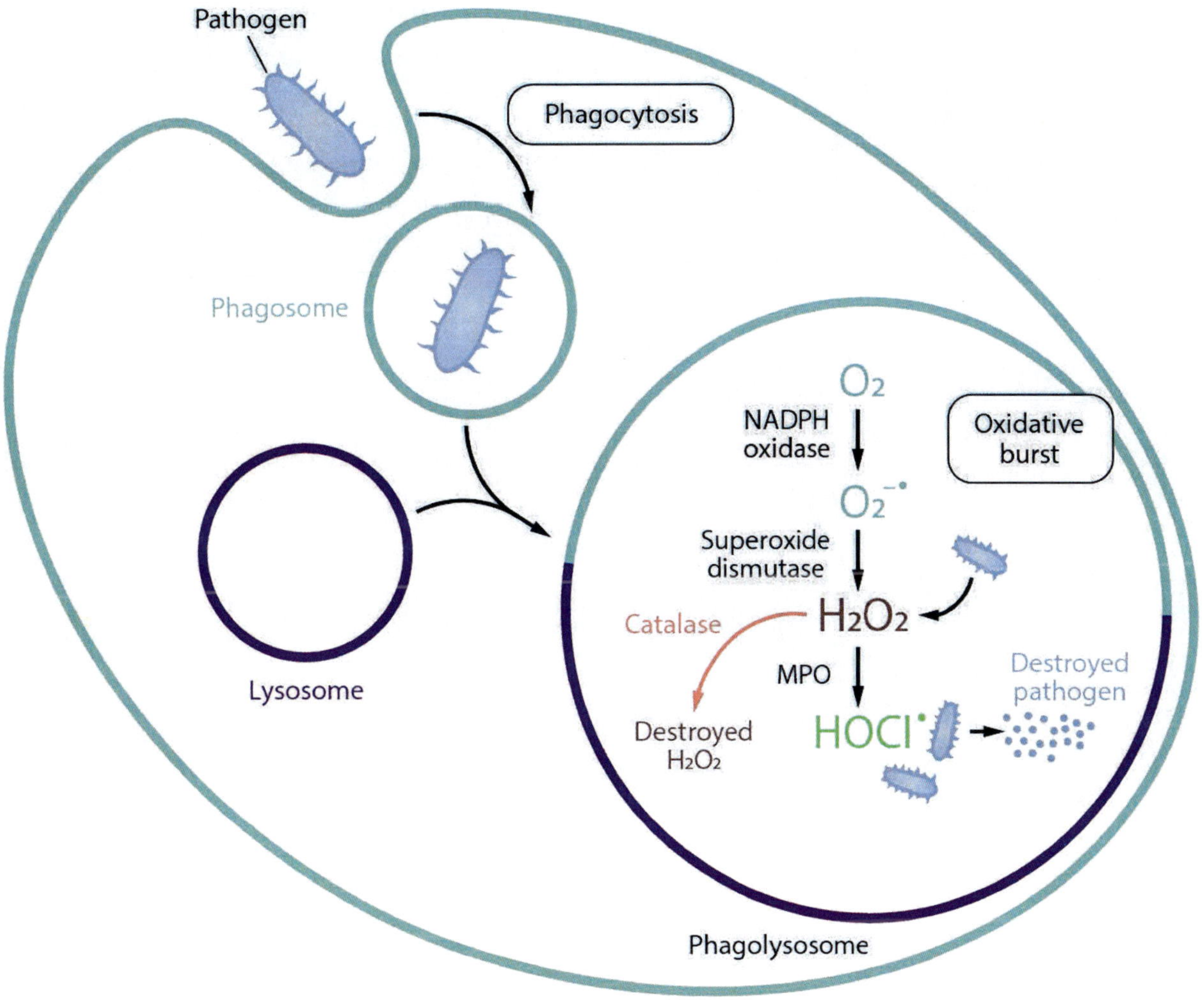

Figure 8.1.17 - Neutrophil phagocytosis and pathogen killing

C. Myeloperoxidase (MPO) converts H_2O_2 to bleach ($HOCl^{\cdot}$, also called hypochlorite) which kills the pathogen

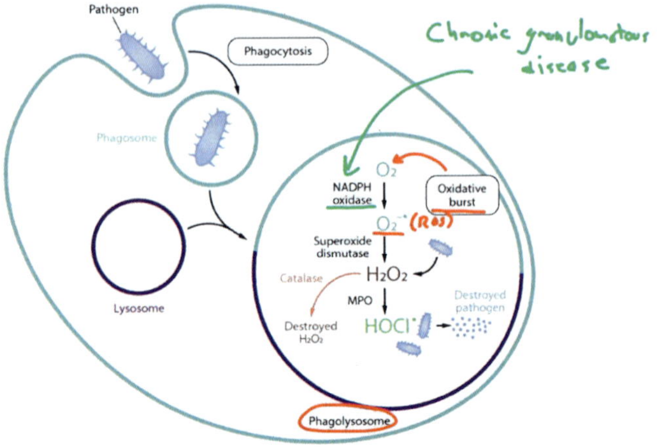

V. Catalase

A. NADPH oxidase is absent in chronic granulomatous disease (CGD)

B. Neutrophils in CGD can kill most bacteria using bacteria-produced H_2O_2

C. Catalase breaks down H_2O_2 → catalase positive organisms leave the phagolysosome without any substrate → pathogen survival

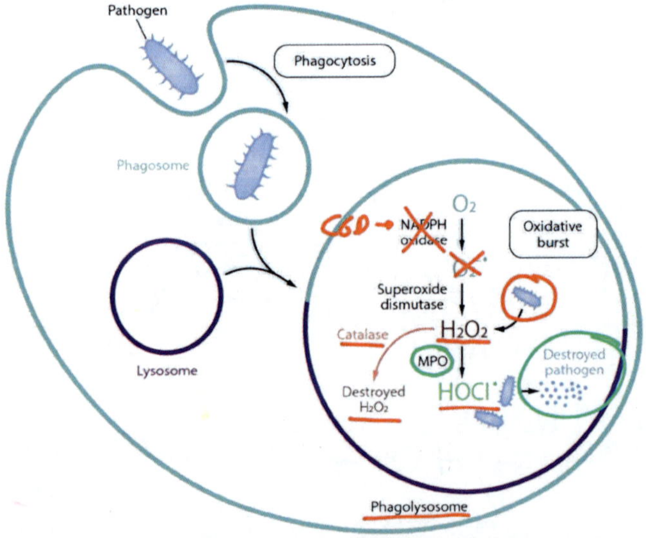

VI. Apoptosis and Pus

A. Performing the oxidative burst depletes energy stores → apoptosis

B. Collection of dead bacteria and neutrophils → pus

REVIEW QUESTIONS

1. The neutrophils in a patient are able to roll along the vascular wall through weak interactions. However, there is a protein deficiency on neutrophils that prevents them from tightly binding to endothelial cells. As a result, the neutrophils continue rolling along the vascular wall without stopping at the site of inflammation. What protein is likely deficient?

- **Correct answer: LFA-1 (CD18)**
- **The question is focused on neutrophil extravasation**
- **Apparently the neutrophils do a fine job performing those weak interactions with the endothelial cells → margination and rolling intact**
- **The inability to tightly bind (adhere) to vascular wall indicates adhesion dysfunction (LFA-1/CD18 on neutrophils vs. ICAM and VCAM on endothelial cells)**
  - **Note: If you thought the answer was PECAM-1, you likely understand the process of extravasation. However, before the neutrophil can utilize PECAM-1 and transmigrate to the inflamed tissue, it must first adhere to the vascular wall. If the neutrophils continue rolling without stopping, we assume they were never able to adhere.**

The neutrophils in a patient are able to roll along the vascular wall through weak interactions. However, there is a protein deficiency on neutrophils that prevents them from tightly binding to endothelial cells. As a result, the neutrophils continue rolling along the vascular wall without stopping at the site of inflammation. What protein is likely deficient?

LFA-1 (CD-18)

Neutrophil extravasation
Margination
Rolling
Tight binding (adhesion)

Section IV - Kinin

I. Kinin System

A. The liver produces 3 proteins relevant to the kinin system that float freely in the blood:

1. Factor XII
2. Prekallikrein
3. High molecular weight kininogen (HMWK)

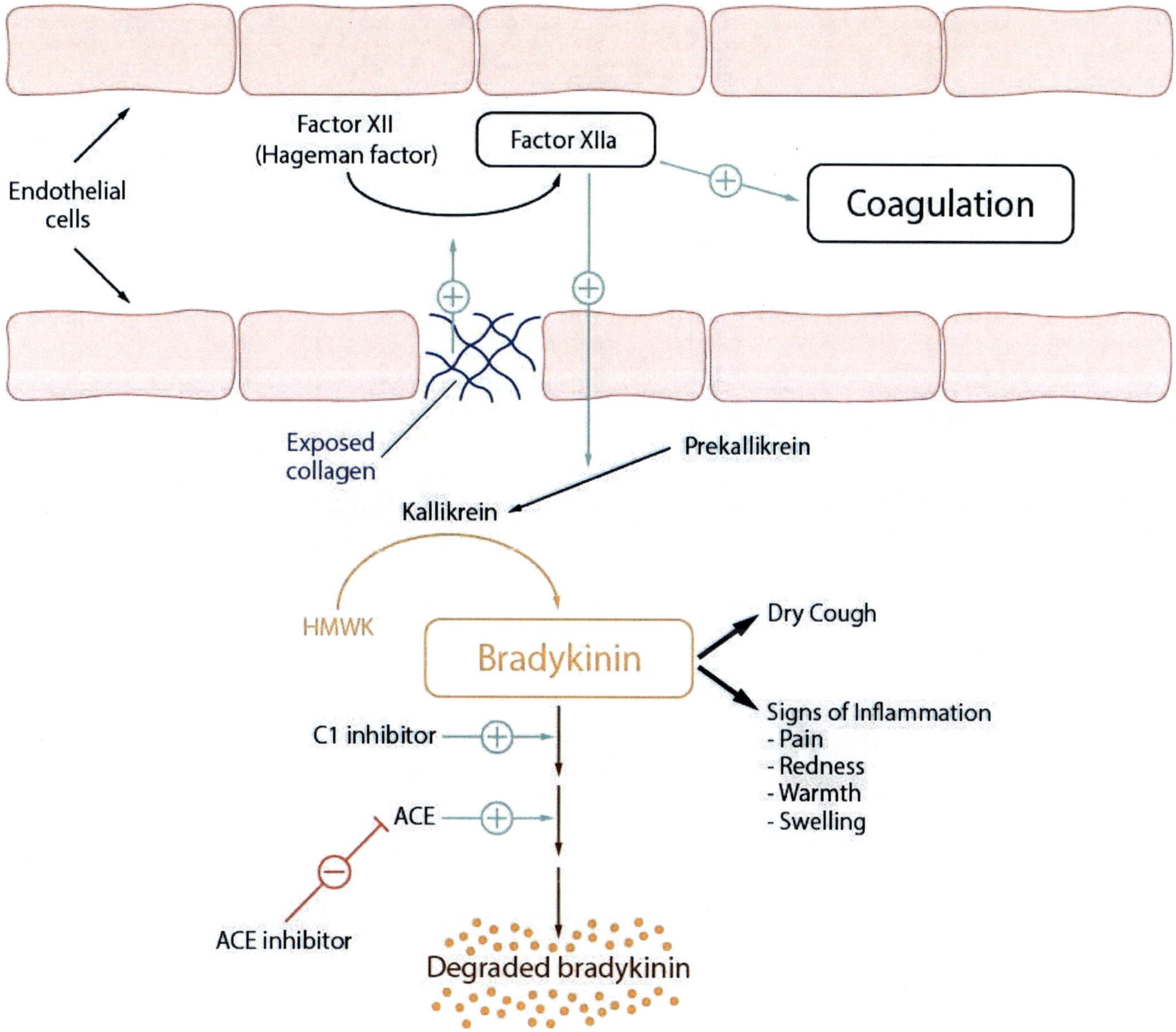

Figure 8.1.18 - Kinin system

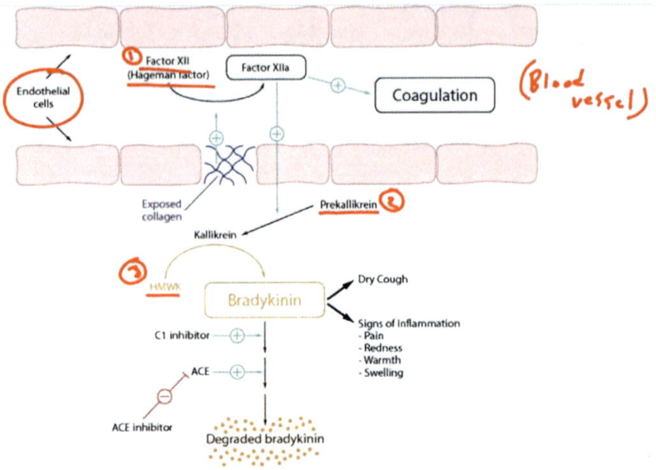

B. Endothelial damage exposes tissue collagen to Factor XII (Hageman factor) → collagen activates Factor XII → activated Factor XII (Factor XIIa) performs 2 roles:

1. Initiates the coagulation cascade (coagulation)
2. Converts prekallikrein to kallikrein (kinin system)

C. Kallikrein converts high molecular weight kininogen (HMWK) to bradykinin

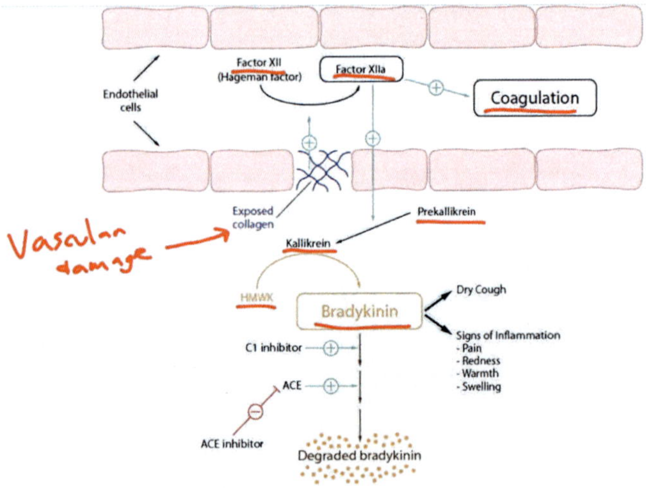

II. Bradykinin Actions

A. Arteriole dilation → redness and warmth
B. ↑ postcapillary permeability → swelling
C. Pain fiber stimulation → pain
D. Smooth muscle constriction of bronchi → dry cough

III. Bradykinin Degradation

A. Bradykinin degradation is upregulated by C1 inhibitor and angiotensin converting enzyme (ACE)

1. C1 inhibitor gets its name from its other role in the complement system

B. C1 inhibitor deficiency (hereditary angioedema) → dangerously high levels of bradykinin

IV. Hereditary Angioedema

A. Pathophysiology: C1 inhibitor deficiency → ↑ bradykinin

B. Presentation: swelling (dangerous angioedema) and dry cough

1. ACE inhibitors worsen angioedema and cough

C. Diagnosis: ↓ C4 levels on lab analysis

1. ↑ C1 activation → more C4 activated to C4a

D. Treatment: C1 inhibitor concentrate

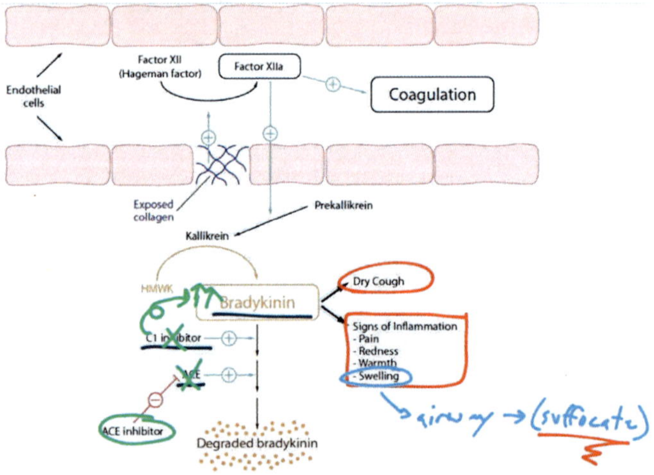

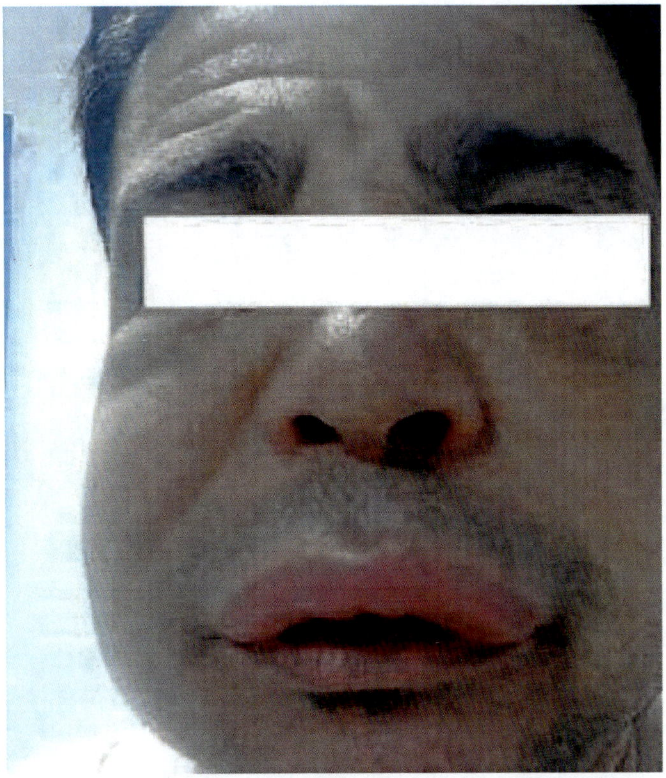

Photo Credit: Boussetta N1*, Ghedira H2, Hamdi MS1, Ariba BY1, Metoui L1, Ghasallah I1, Zriba S2, Louzir B1, Msaddak F2, Ajili F1 and Othmani S11 - Department of Internal Medicine, Military Hospital of Tunis, Tunisia2 - Department of Hematology, Military Hospital of Tunis, Tunisia [CC BY 4.0 (https://creativecommons.org/licenses/by/4.0)]

Figure 8.1.19 - Angioedema

REVIEW QUESTIONS

1. A patient steps on a thumb tack which causes her to bleed. As a result of this insult, bradykinin is produced and the coagulation cascade is initiated. What is the immediate precursor to bradykinin? How does the kinin system relate to the coagulation cascade?

   - **Correct answer: HMWK; Hageman factor (factor XIIa) is where kinin and coagulation intersect**
   - **Damage to vascular wall → interstitial collagen exposed → factor XII (Hageman factor) gets activated to factor XIIa → factor XIIa initiates coagulation and converts prekallikrein to kallikrein**
   - **Kallikrein then converts HMWK to bradykinin (ie, the immediate precursor to bradykinin is HMWK)**

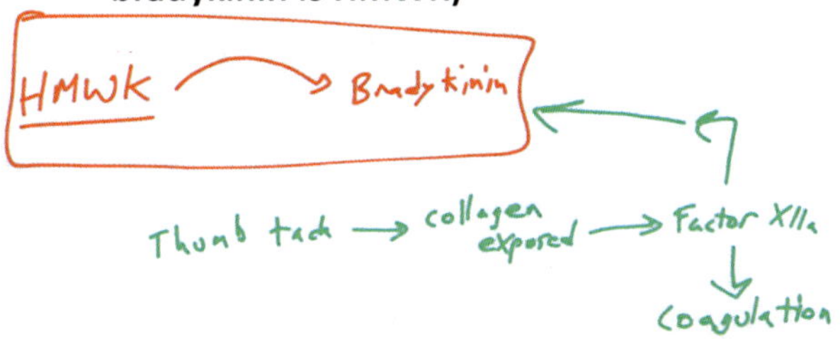

Section V - Complement

I. Complement System Overview

A. Composed of plasma proteins synthesized in the liver

B. When activated, these proteins will form complexes that complement acute inflammation (eg, neutrophil chemotaxis, mast cell degranulation, etc)

II. Three possible ways to initiate the complement system:

A. Spontaneous (alternative)

B. Lectin

C. Classic

D. All 3 pathways lead to the formation of a C3 convertase

E. General flow: C3 convertase → C5 convertase → membrane attack complex (MAC)

1. MAC is especially important for lysis of encapsulated bacteria

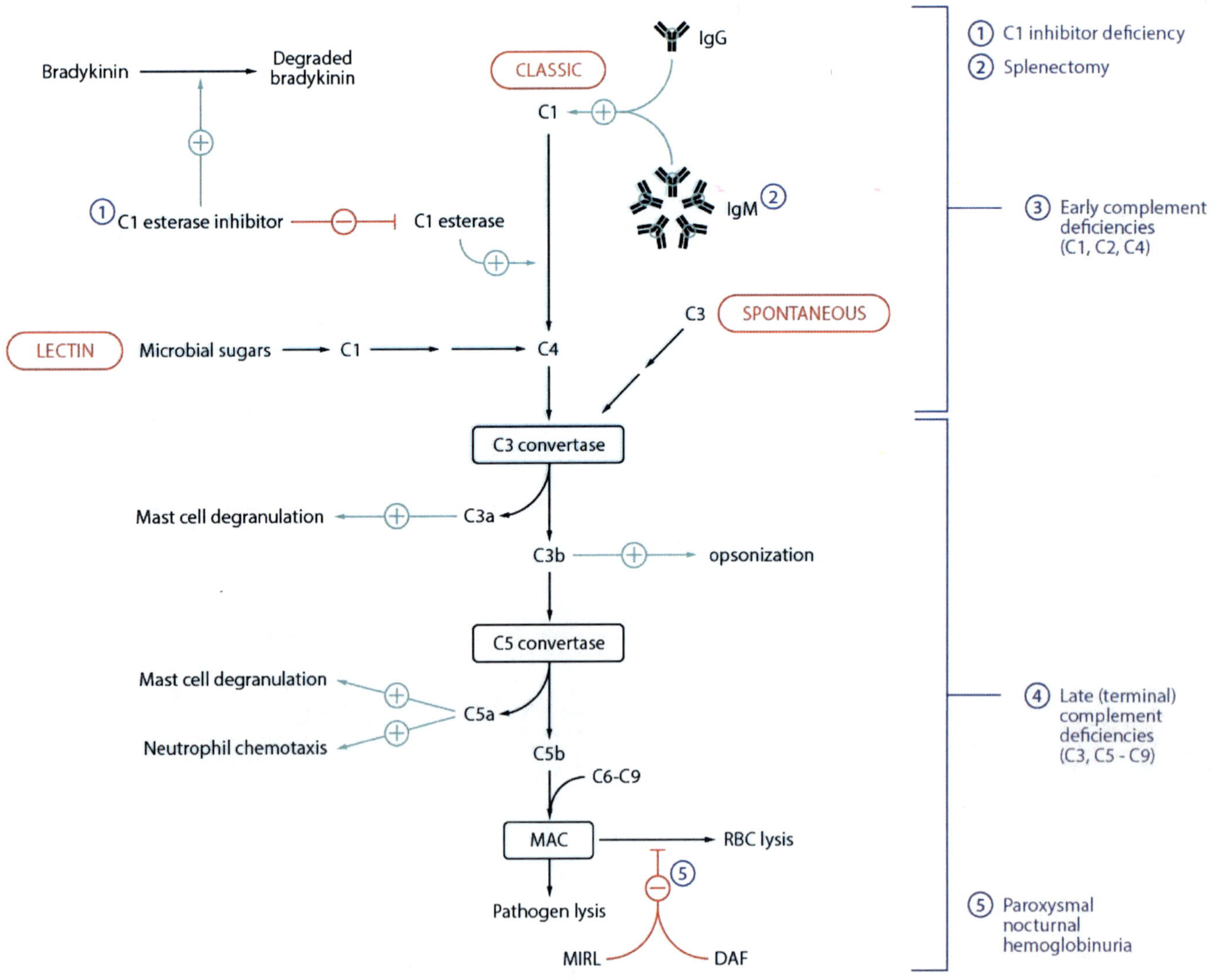

Figure 8.1.20 - Complement system and deficiencies

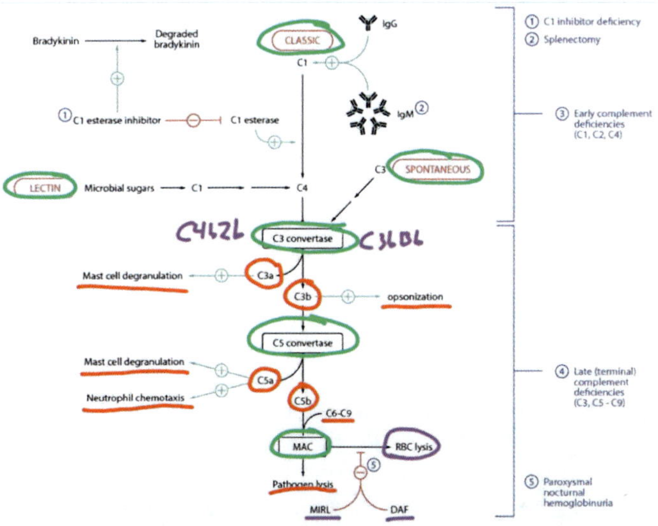

Disease	Problem	Description	Clinical Notes
Early complement deficiencies (C1, C2, or C4)	- A group of diseases characterized by a deficiency in one or more early complement proteins	- Failure to lyse encapsulated organisms - C1, C2, and C4 proteins are required to clear immune complexes → immune complex persistence can lead to SLE	- Recurrent infections of encapsulated bacteria (H. influenzae type b, S. pneumoniae, N. meningitidis) - High risk of SLE
Late (terminal) complement deficiencies (C3 or C5-C9)	- A group of diseases characterized by a deficiency in one or more late complement proteins	- Failure to lyse encapsulated organisms	- Recurrent infections of encapsulated bacteria (especially N. meningitidis)
Splenectomy (asplenia)	- ↓ Macrophage phagocytosis of pathogens - ↓ IgM synthesis which is normally required to fix complement via the classical pathway	- The spleen is a major site of macrophage phagocytosis of encapsulated organisms as well as IgM synthesis - Loss of splenic macrophages → ↓ ability to destroy encapsulated organisms - Loss of IgM-mediated complement fixation → ↓ ability to destroy encapsulated organisms	- Recurrent infections of encapsulated bacteria (H. influenzae type b, S. pneumoniae, N. meningitidis)
Hereditary angioedema	- C1 inhibitor deficiency	- C1 inhibitor has two roles: promote complement activation and breakdown of bradykinin - Deficient C1 inhibitor → ↑ bradykinin → angioedema - Deficient C1 inhibitor → ↑ conversion of C4 to C4a	- Angioedema - ↓ C4 levels - Treat with C1 inhibitor concentrate - Avoid ACE inhibitors
Paroxysmal nocturnal hemoglobinuria	- Inability to prevent complement-mediated red blood cell (RBC) lysis	- RBCs normally prevent formation of MAC on their surface via DAF/CD55 and MIRL/CD59 which are anchored to the RBC via GPI proteins - Mutations in the PIGA gene results in a lack of GPI anchor proteins expressed on RBC membranes → lack of DAF/CD55 and MIRL/CD59 → RBC lysis	- Anemia - ↓ haptoglobin - Dark urine

Table 8.1.2 - Complement deficiencies

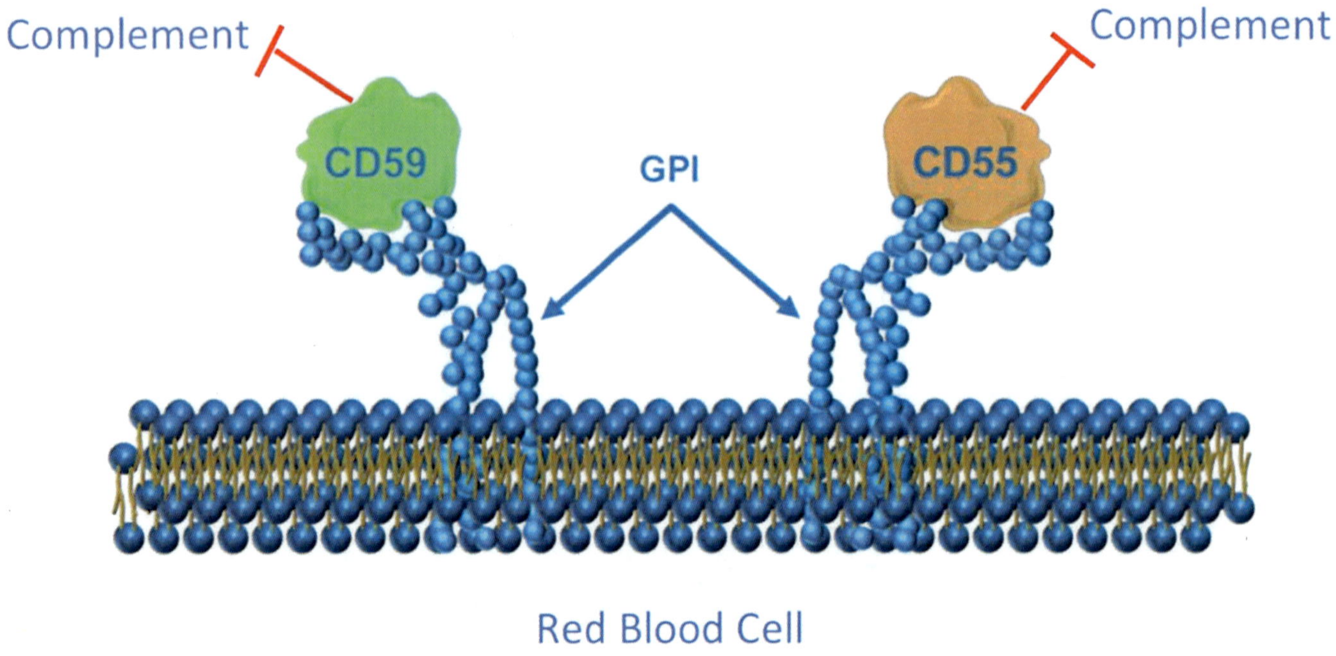

Figure 8.1.21 - CD59 and CD55

REVIEW QUESTIONS

1. A 40-year-old female patient lacks sufficient levels of a certain complement protein. She also has systemic lupus erythematosus. She will be most susceptible to which specific pathogen(s)?

   - **Correct answer: This patient has an early complement deficiency.**
   - **Insufficient levels of C1, C2, and C4 → inability to adequately clear immune complexes → increased risk of SLE, as seen in this patient**
   - **Low serum C1, C2 or C4 indicates an early complement deficiency → increased susceptibility to infection with 3 encapsulated organisms: H. influenzae type b, S. pneumoniae, and N. meningitidis**
     - **Note: If you were thinking she would only be susceptible to N. meningitidis, you were likely thinking of late complement deficiencies (remember that patients with late complement deficiencies are not likely to get lupus because levels of C1, C2, and C4 are sufficient)**

Early complement def. → ↓MAC → H.flu. b, S.pneumo, N. men.
↓
low C1, C2, C4
↓
HIGH immune complexes → SLE

Section VI - Chronic Inflammation

I. Chronic Inflammation Overview

A. Definition:

1. Delayed inflammatory response that includes elements from innate and adaptive immunity

B. Causes:

1. Prolonged infection (most common), autoimmune disease (eg, SLE), or reaction to foreign agent (eg, silica)

C. Morphology:

1. Lymphocyte infiltration (mainly activated T cells)

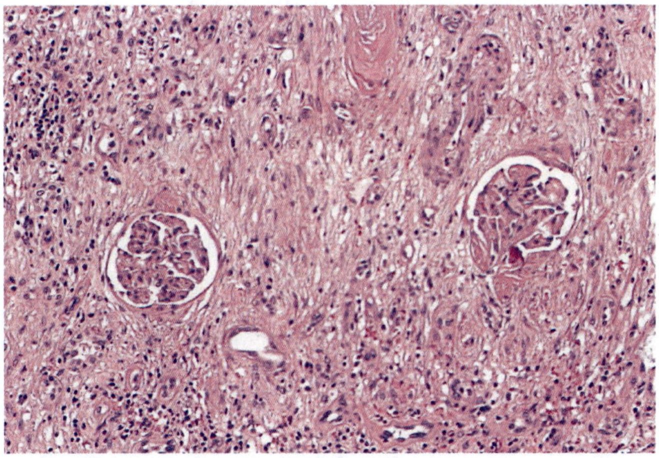

Figure 8.1.23 - Lymphocytic infiltration on tissue biopsy

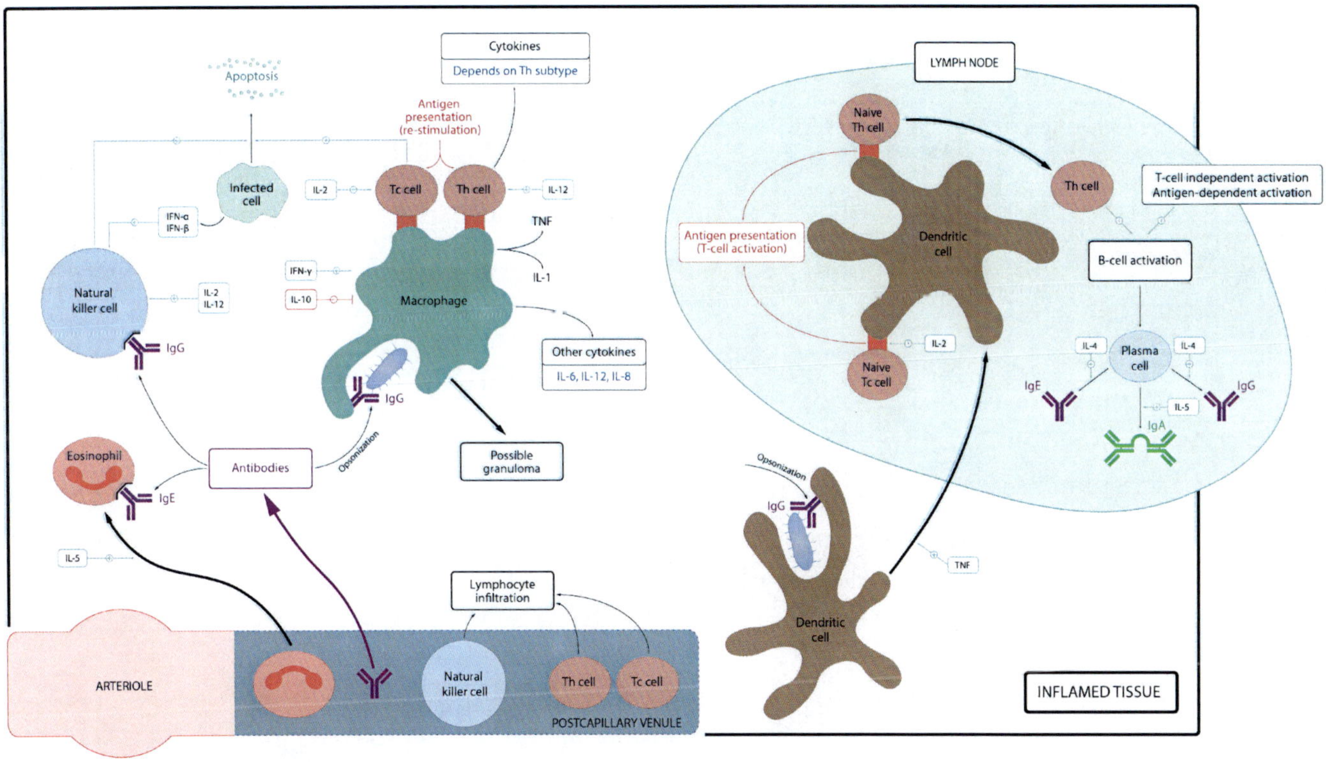

Figure 8.1.22 - Chronic inflammation overview

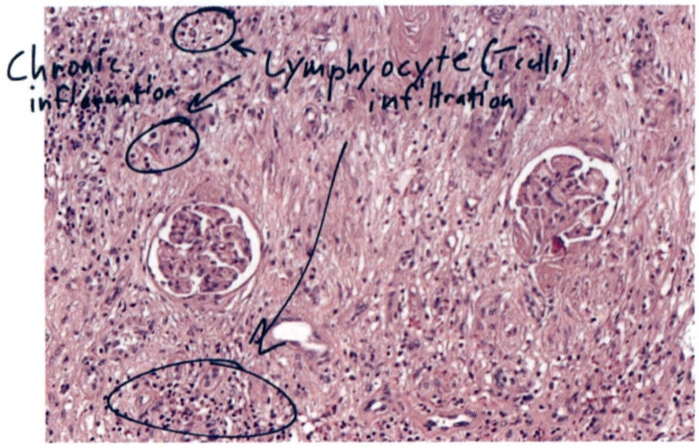

II. Chronic Inflammation Timeline

- A. T-cell activation
  1. Dendritic cells travel
  2. Antigen presentation
  3. T cell and B cell activation
- B. Lymphocyte infiltration
- C. Cellular activities (NK, Tc, Th, macrophages, eosinophils)
- D. Antibody influence on cellular activities
- E. Granulomas

III. T-cell Activation

- A. Dendritic cells travel
  1. After phagocytosis, dendritic cells will travel from acutely inflamed tissue to local lymph nodes
- B. Antigen presentation and activation
  1. Once in lymph nodes, dendritic cells will present antigens to naive T cells → naive helper T cells and naive cytotoxic T cells become activated
- C. T cell and B cell activation
  1. Following activation, helper T cells will activate B cells → plasma cells will release antibodies from lymphoid organs

IV. Lymphocyte Infiltration

- A. Lymphocytes will marginate, roll, adhere and transmigrate toward the site of inflammation much like neutrophils
- B. The predominant lymphocytes that infiltrate tissues in chronic inflammation are activated T cells (Tc and Th)

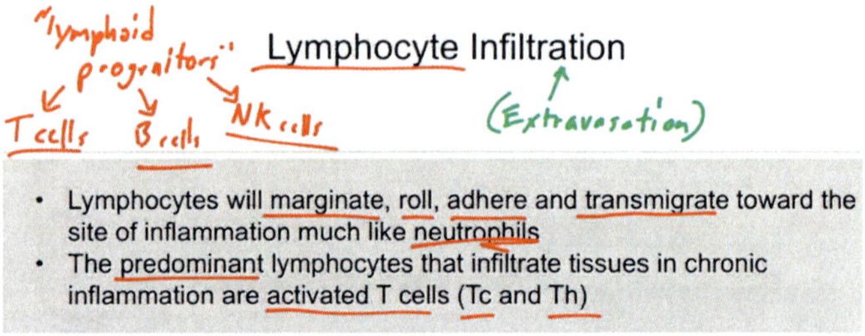

V. Helper T Cells

- A. Helper T cells come in 4 subtypes:
  1. Th1
  2. Th2
  3. Th17
  4. Treg
- B. The cytokines released from helper T cells depends on the subtype

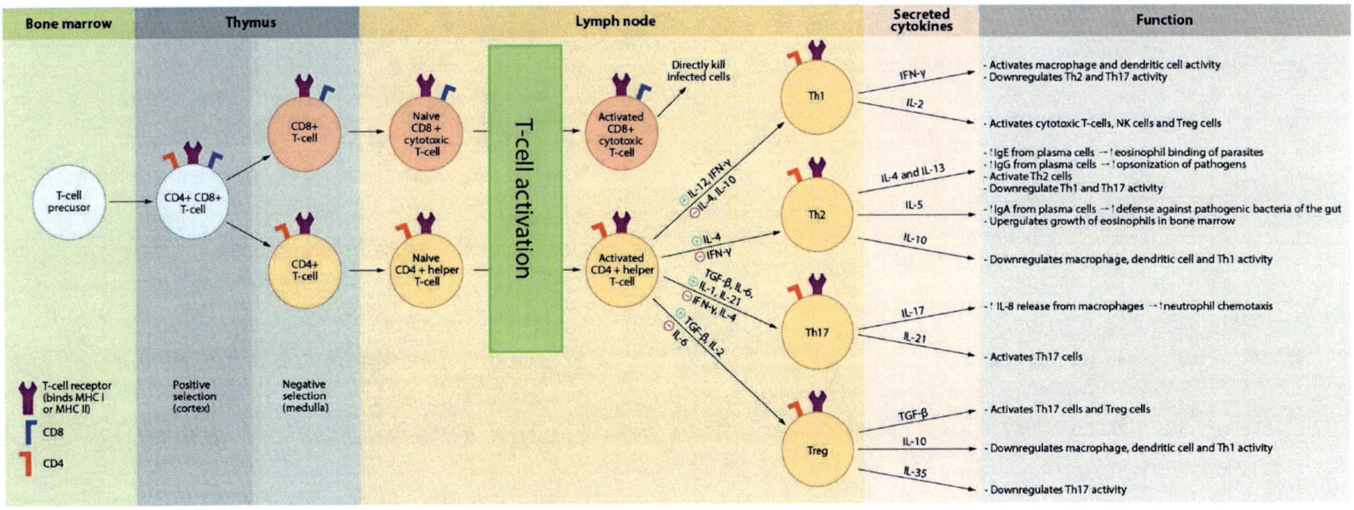

Figure 8.1.24 - T-cell differentiation and maturation

VI. Macrophages in Chronic Inflammation

A. Remain local and perform phagocytosis and antigen presentation in the inflamed tissue → re-stimulation of already activated helper T cells and cytotoxic T cells

B. Macrophages release IL-1 and TNF which perpetuate inflammation

C. Other cytokines that macrophages release depend on what activities are needed

1. IL-6 → fever and ↑ Th17 activity
2. IL-8 → neutrophil chemotaxis
3. IL-12 → ↑ Th1 and NK cell activity

VII. Eosinophils

A. Important in defense against parasites

B. Th2 cells increase eosinophil activity in 2 ways:

1. IL-5 release → ↑ eosinophil production in the bone marrow
2. IL-4 release → ↑ IgE-releasing plasma cells

C. IgE will bind to parasites (esp. helminths) → eosinophils will bind to Fc portion of IgE and release major basic protein (MBP) → destruction of helminth

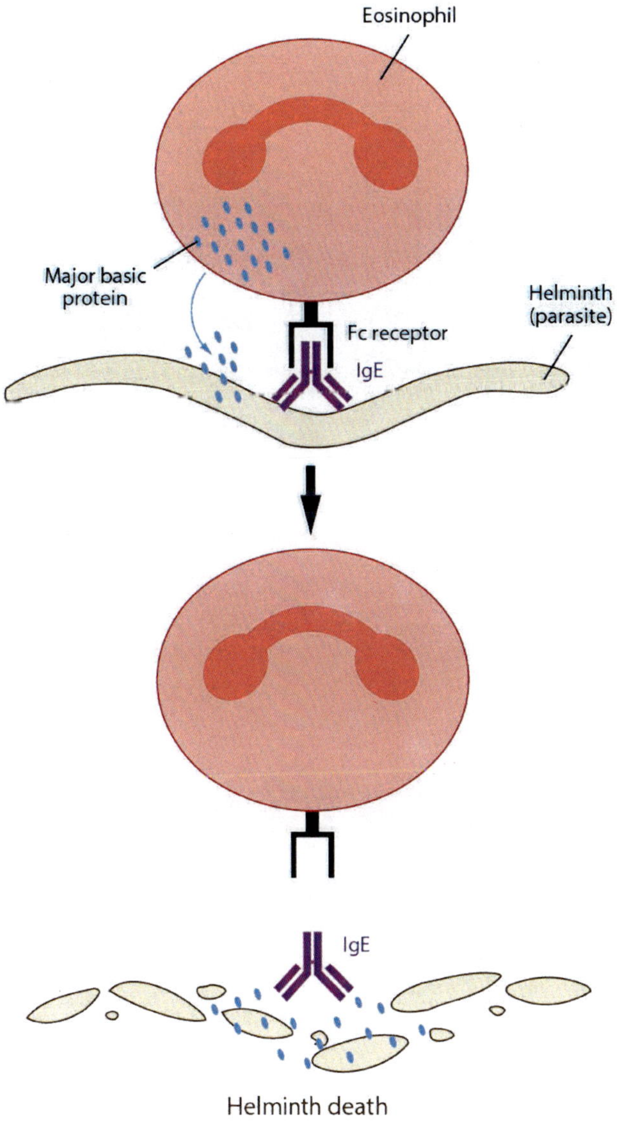

Figure 8.1.25 - IgE-mediated activation of eosinophils

VIII. Antibodies in Inflammation

A. Antibodies will bind to pathogen

B. IgG-bound pathogens

1. ↑ opsonization and phagocytosis by macrophages and dendritic cells

2. ↑ activity of natural killer cells

C. IgE-bound pathogens (parasites)

D. ↑ activity of eosinophils

REVIEW QUESTIONS ?

1. A 22-year-old male presents to the emergency department 3 weeks after being stabbed in the leg. He was initially hesitant to present to a clinician because he was embarrassed for getting into a knife fight at a bar. On physical examination, the wounded area is swollen and tender to the touch. There doesn't appear to be any indication of pus. What are the predominant immune cells at the site of injury? Where were these cells initially activated?

   - **Correct answer: T cells; lymph nodes**
   - **The lack of pus indicates the inflammation is not acute**
   - **Chronic inflammation is marked by lymphocytic (T-cell infiltration)**
   - **T-cells are initially activated in lymph nodes by dendritic cells, and then travel to the site of inflammation**

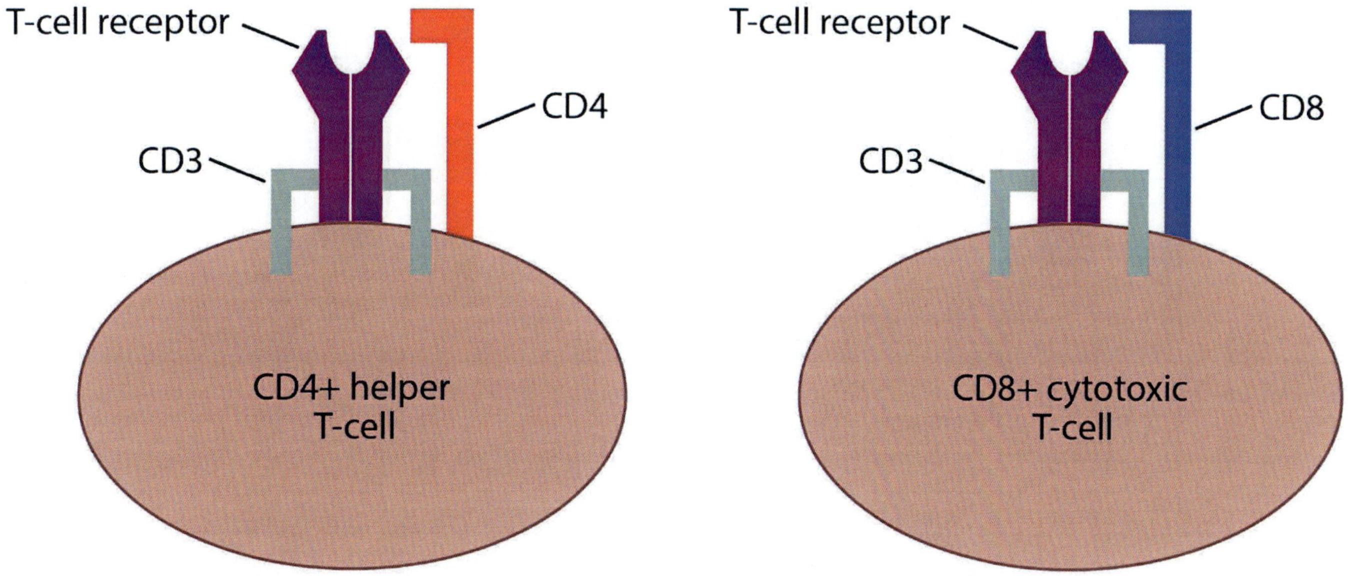

Figure 8.1.26 - CD4+ helper T-cell and CD8+ cytotoxic T-cell

I. T-cells
   A. T-cell receptor binds to MHC
   B. CD3 transmits signal intracellularly
   C. CD4 → T-helper cells
      1. Many functions (eg, stimulate B-cells to make antibodies, produce cytokines)
   D. CD8 → cytotoxic T-cells
      1. Directly kill cells

II. Major Histocompatibility Complexes (MHCs)
   A. MHCs: protein structures that present antigen fragments to T-cell receptors
   B. Encoded by HLA genes
   C. 2 important classes:
      1. MHC class I
      2. MHC class II

	MHC I	MHC II
Structure	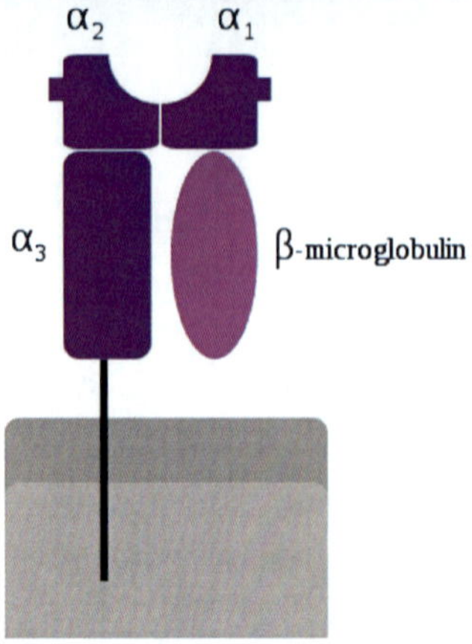 1 long chain made of α subunits 1 short chain known as β2 microglobulin	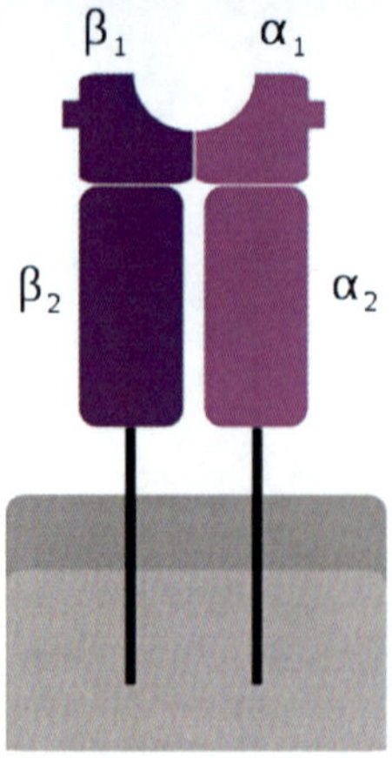 2 chains of equal length 2 α subunits and 2 β subunits
Expression	All nucleated cells as well as platelets and APCs	APCs only
Function	Present intracellular antigens to CD8+ T-cells (cytotoxic T-cells)	Present extracellular antigens to CD4+ T-cells (T helper cells)
Binds	CD8 and T-cell receptors	CD4 and T-cell receptors
Antigen loading	Protein degraded to peptides by proteasome. TAP delivers peptides to the RER where they are loaded onto MHC I.	Invariant chain added first and cleaved to form CLIP. CLIP removed in acidified endosome where antigen replaces it.
Genetic loci	HLA-A, HLA-B, HLA-C	HLA-DP, HLA-DQ, HLA-DR

Table 8.1.3 - MHC I and MHC II

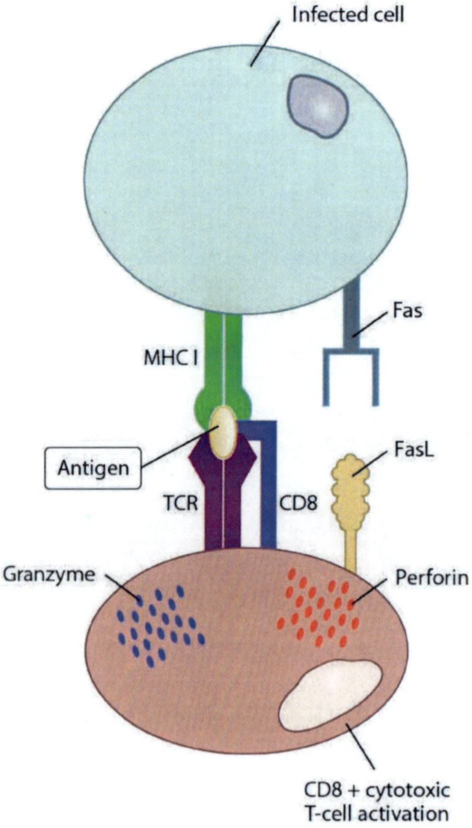

Figure 8.1.27 - CD8+ cytotoxic T-cell activation

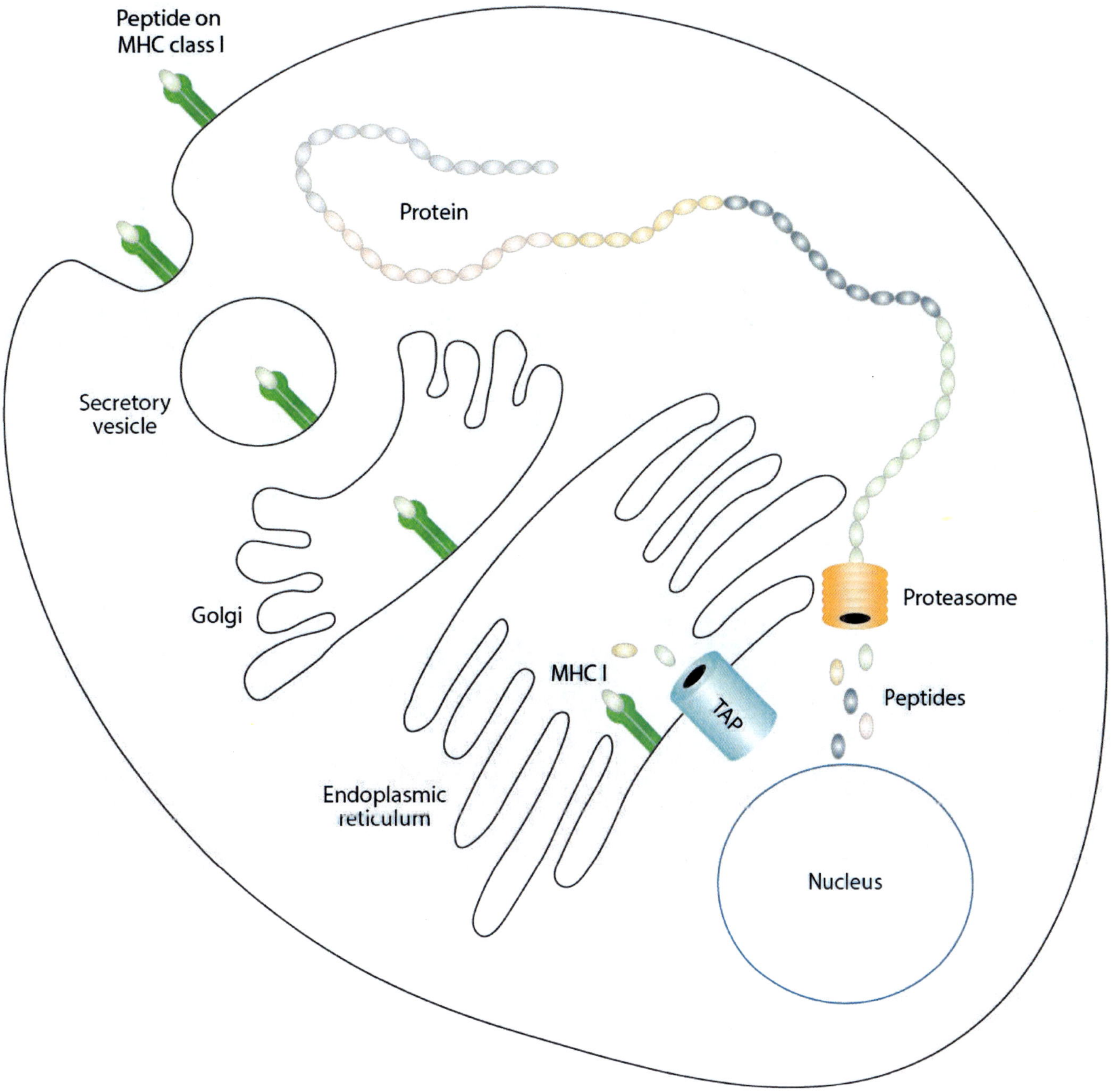

Figure 8.1.28 - Antigen presentation on MHC I

III. Bare Lymphocyte Syndrome

  A. Mutation in genes encoding for TAP

  B. Absence of MHC class I

  C. Impaired cytotoxic T-cell activity

  D. Normal lymphocyte count

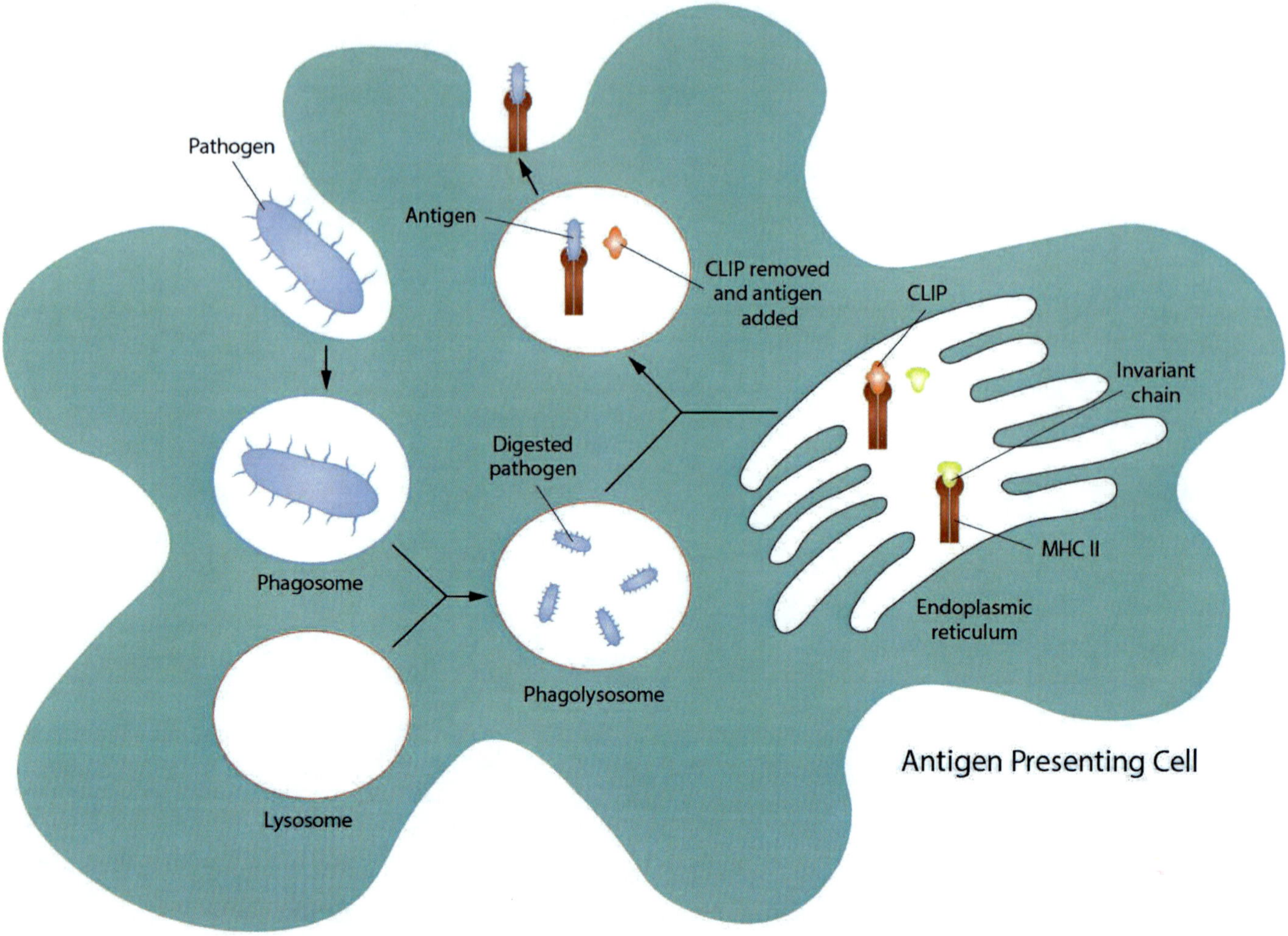

Figure 8.1.29 - Antigen presentation on MHC II

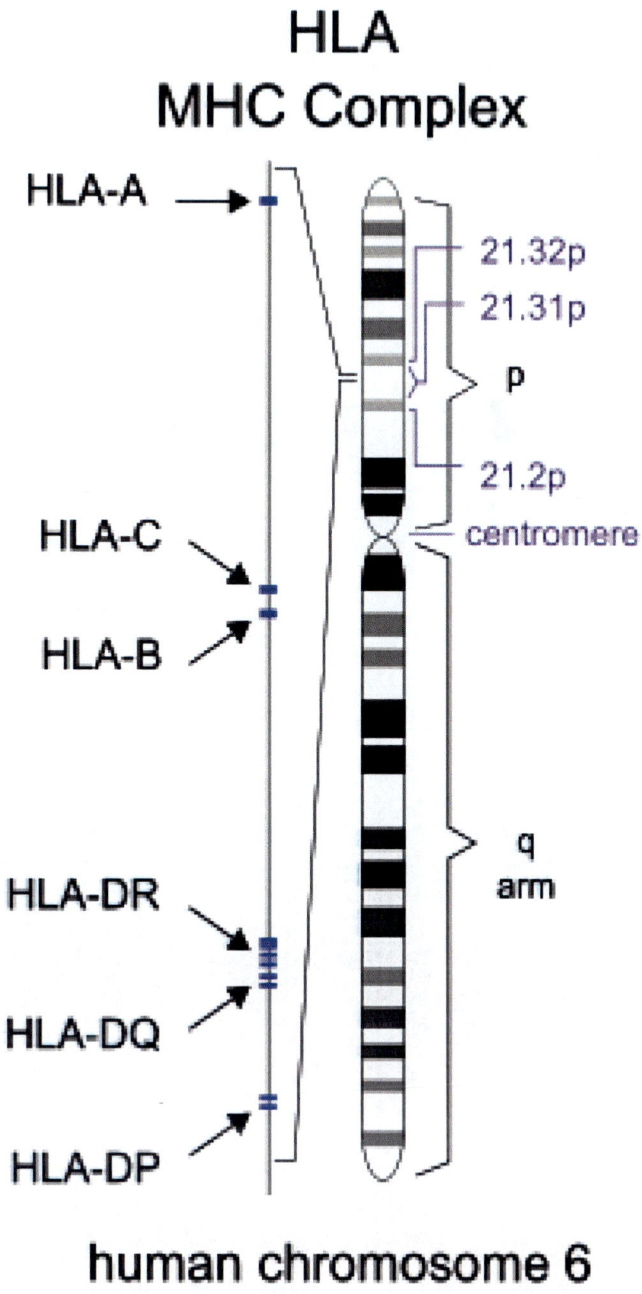

Photo Credit: HLA.jpg: Pdeitiker at en.wikipediaderivative work: Faigl.ladislav

Figure 8.1.30 - HLA genes

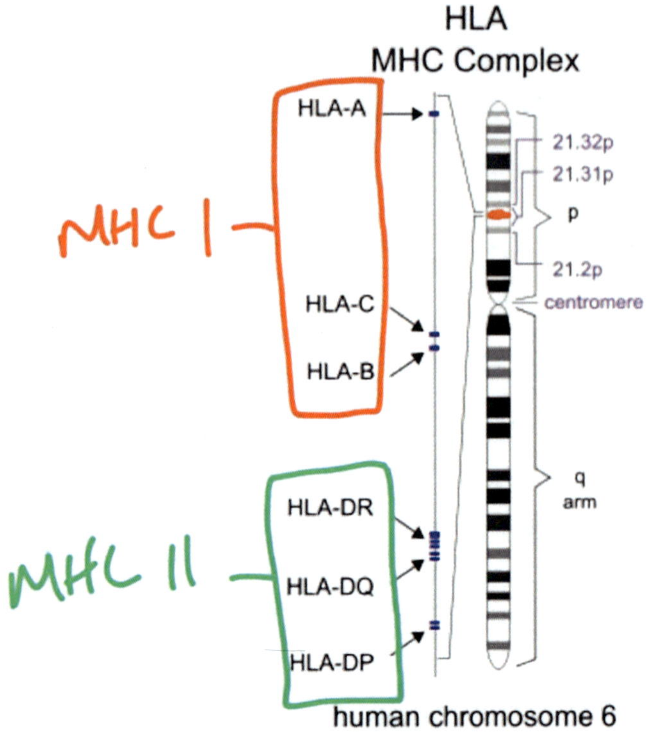

IV. HLA Subtype Associations - MHC I

A. HLA-A3 - hemochromatosis

B. HLA-B8 - Addison's disease, myasthenia gravis, Graves' disease

C. HLA-B27 - psoriatic arthritis, ankylosing spondylitis, IBD-associated arthritis, reactive arthritis

D. HLA-C - psoriasis

V. HLA Subtype Associations - MHC II

A. HLA-DQ2/HLA-DQ8 - celiac disease

B. HLA-DR2 - multiple sclerosis, hay fever, SLE, Goodpasture's syndrome

C. HLA-DR3 - DM type I, SLE, Graves' disease, Hashimoto's thyroiditis, Addison's disease

D. HLA-DR4 - rheumatoid arthritis, DM type 1, Addison's disease

E. HLA-DR5 - Hashimoto's thyroiditis

REVIEW QUESTIONS ?

1. Researchers are studying the effects of knockout mutations of the gene associated with the invariant chain that is normally loaded onto MHC class II molecules. A defect in the invariant chain would most likely result in the presentation of what type of antigens?

- **The answer to the question is self antigens.**
- **The MHC II complex is synthesized in the rough ER along with many other proteins.**
- **The invariant chain normally prevents self antigens from being loaded onto the MHC II complex.**
- **If the invariant chain were defective, then the proteins synthesized in the rough ER could be loaded onto the MHC II complex and the antigen presenting cell would present self-antigens.**

Section VIII - Macrophages

I. Macrophage Activities Overview
   A. Acute inflammation
      1. Infiltrates tissue within 2-3 days
      2. Phagocytosis and O2-independent killing
      3. Cytokine secretion
      4. Possible abscess formation
   B. Chronic inflammation
      1. Local antigen presentation
      2. Cytokine secretion
      3. Possible granuloma formation

II. Macrophage Phagocytosis
   A. Phagocytosis
      1. Identifies what cells to engulf
      2. Enhanced by opsonins

III. Surface Proteins in Phagocytosis
   A. CD14 (a TLR) → binds to PAMPs (eg, LPS) and DAMPs (eg, necrotic tissue)
   B. Fc receptor → binds to IgG (opsonin)
   C. C3b receptor → binds to C3b (opsonin)

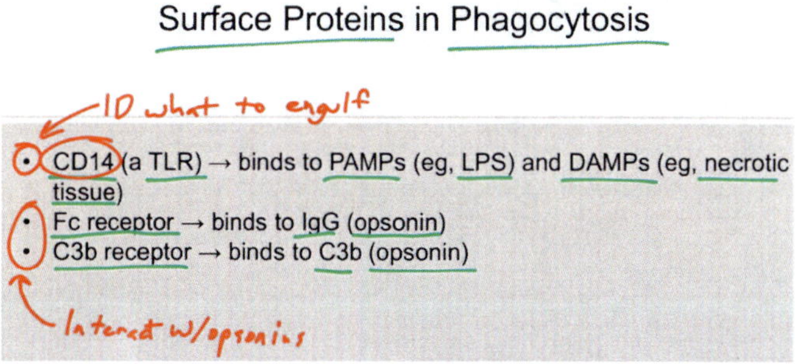
Surface Proteins in Phagocytosis

ID what to engulf

- CD14 (a TLR) → binds to PAMPs (eg, LPS) and DAMPs (eg, necrotic tissue)
- Fc receptor → binds to IgG (opsonin)
- C3b receptor → binds to C3b (opsonin)

Interact w/opsonins

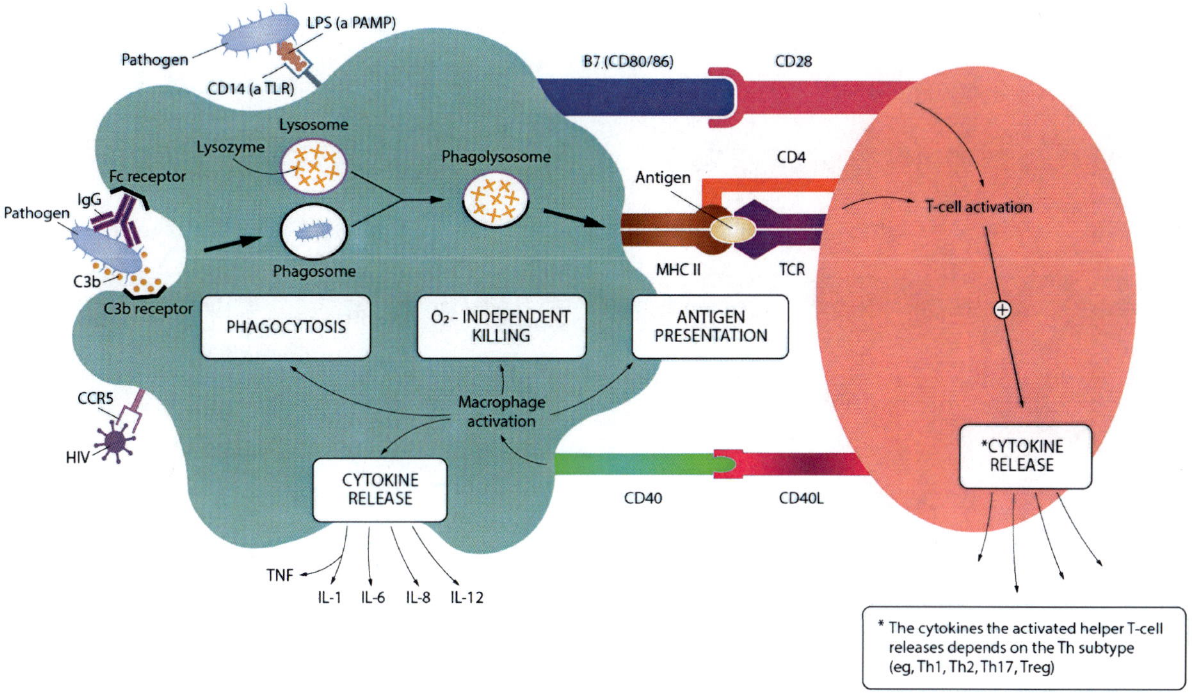

Figure 8.1.31 - Macrophage interaction with T cell

IV. Macrophage O_2-independent Killing

A. Following phagocytosis, macrophages use lysozyme → hydrolyzes bacterial peptidoglycan → lysis of bacteria

Cell	Cytokine	Function
Macrophages and Dendritic Cells	IL-1	- ↑ prostaglandin production → pain, fever, swelling, redness, warmth - ↑ E-selectins, ICAM, and VCAM on endothelial cells - Activates Th17 cells
	TNF	- ↑ prostaglandin production → pain, fever, swelling, redness, warmth - ↑ E-selectins, ICAM, and VCAM on endothelial cells - Stimulates dendritic cells to enter lymph nodes - Cachexia in malignancy - Granuloma maintenance (eg, TB)
	IL-6	- ↑ prostaglandin production in hypothalamus → fever - ↑ release of acute phase proteins - Activates Th17 cells - Downregulates Treg cells
	IL-8	- Neutrophil chemotaxis
	IL-12	- Activates NK cells - Activates Th1 cells

Table 8.1.4 - Cytokines released from macrophages and dendritic cells

V. Abscess Formation

A. Definition:

1. Neutrophils and pus surrounded by a wall of fibrosis

B. Process:

1. Macrophages stimulate fibroblasts

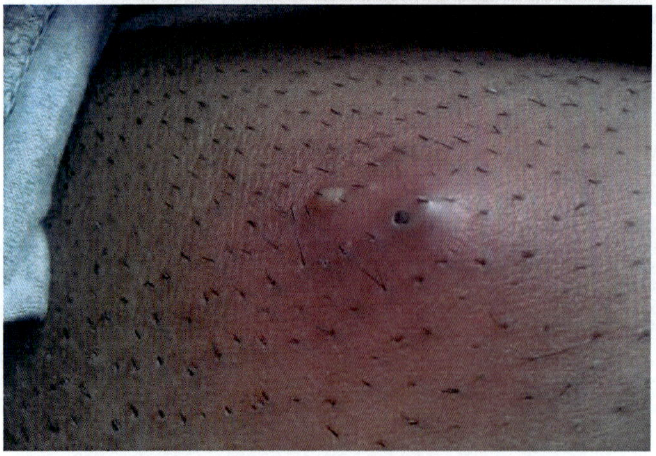

Photo Credit: Amrith Raj [CC BY-SA 3.0 (https://creativecommons.org/licenses/by-sa/3.0)]

Figure 8.1.32 - Abscess

C. Macrophages Antigen Presentation

D. After phagocytosis and oxygen-independent killing, macrophages present antigens locally to activated T cells → re-stimulation of activated T cells

VI. Surface Proteins in Antigen Presentation

A. MHC II and B7 (CD80/86) → helper T-cell restimulation

B. MHC I and B7 (CD80/86) → cytotoxic T-cell restimulation

C. CD40 → macrophage stimulation → continued phagocytosis, O2-independent killing, and antigen presentation

1. Cytokine secretion depends on the helper T-cell subtype (eg, stimulated Th1 cells release IFN-γ which will then stimulate the macrophage to release more IL-12)

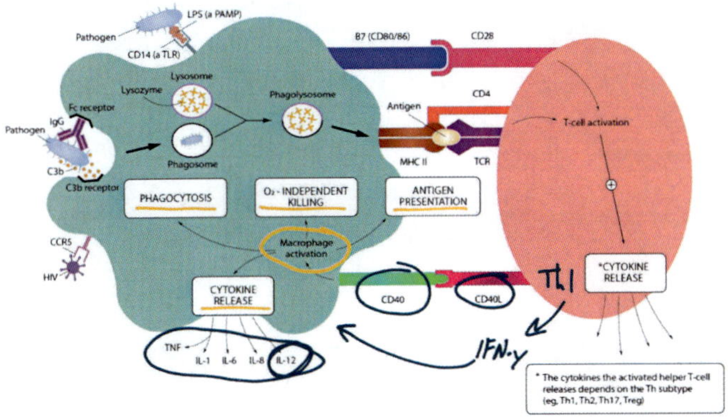

VII. Macrophage Surface Proteins

A. Surface protein targeted by HIV

1. CCR5

VIII. Granulomas

A. Chronic inflammation can be subdivided into two types:

1. Nongranulomatous

2. Granulomatous

a) Caseating

b) Noncaseating

IX. Noncaseating Granulomas

A. Formation

1. Th1 cells release IFN-γ → macrophages become epithelioid cells (aka epithelioid histiocytes) → some epithelioid cells with combine to form multinucleated giant cells → epithelioid and giant cells surround infection → granuloma

B. Appearance

1. Collection of giant cells and epithelioid cells (ovoid nuclei surrounded by lots of pink cytoplasm)

2. Surrounded by lymphocytes (Th1 cells)

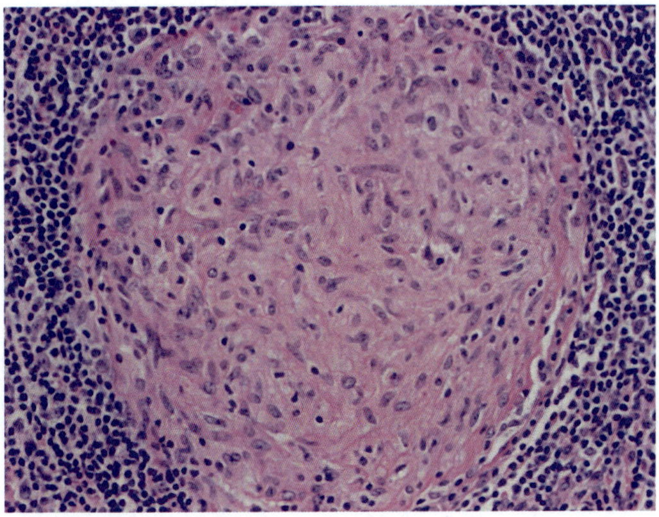

Photo Credit: Sanjay Mukhopadhyay [Public domain]

Figure 8.1.33 - Noncaseating granuloma without a giant cell

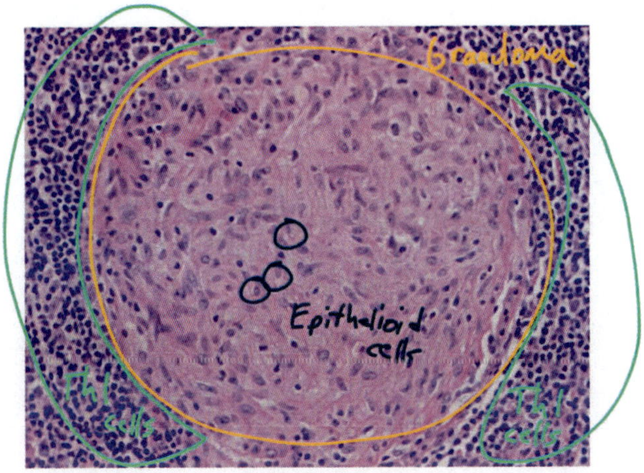

Sanjay Mukhopadhyay [Public domain]

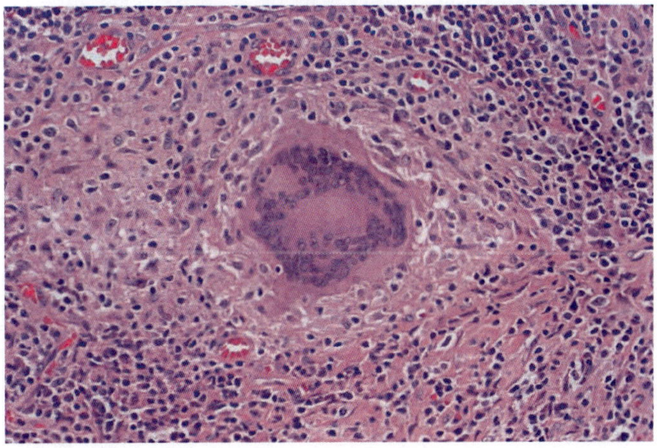

Photo Credit: Ed Uthman via Flickr (CC BY 2.0)

Figure 8.1.34 - Noncaseating granuloma with a giant cell

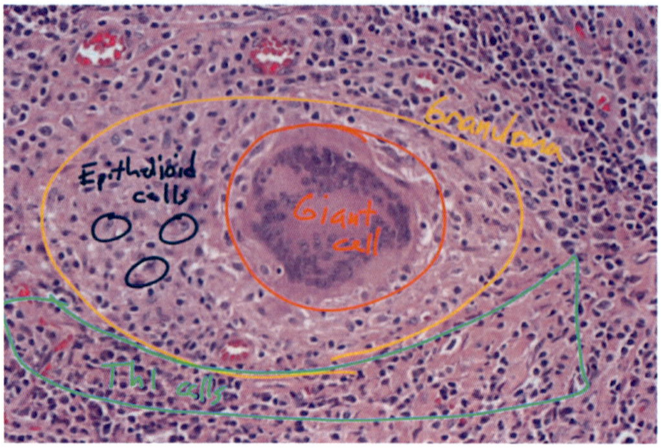

X. Caseating Granulomas

A. Formation

1. Same as noncaseating granulomas

B. Appearance

1. Same as noncaseating granulomas + caseation

2. Caseation: central necrosis (cells lack nuclei) → indicates TB or systemic mycoses (Histoplasmosis, Blastomycosis, Coccidiomycosis, Paracoccidioidomycosis)

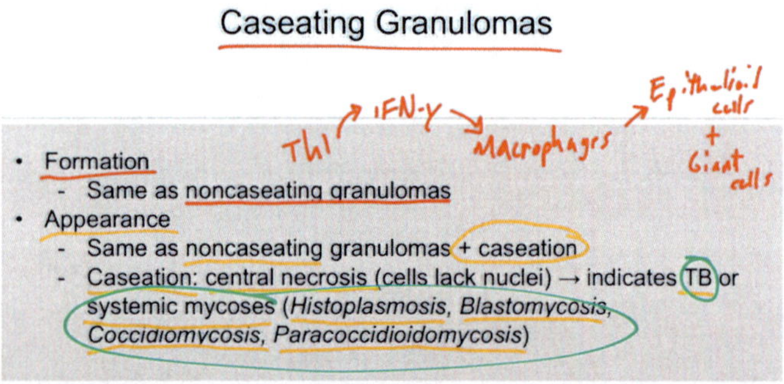
Caseating Granulomas

- Formation
  - Same as noncaseating granulomas
- Appearance
  - Same as noncaseating granulomas + caseation
  - Caseation: central necrosis (cells lack nuclei) → indicates TB or systemic mycoses (*Histoplasmosis*, *Blastomycosis*, *Coccidiomycosis*, *Paracoccidioidomycosis*)

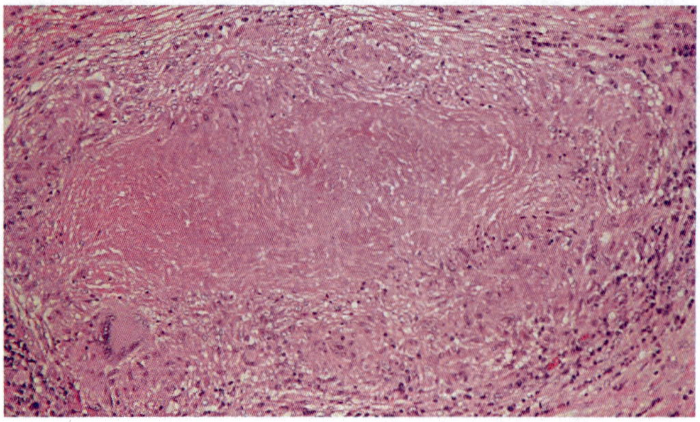

Figure 8.1.35 - Caseating granuloma with a giant cell

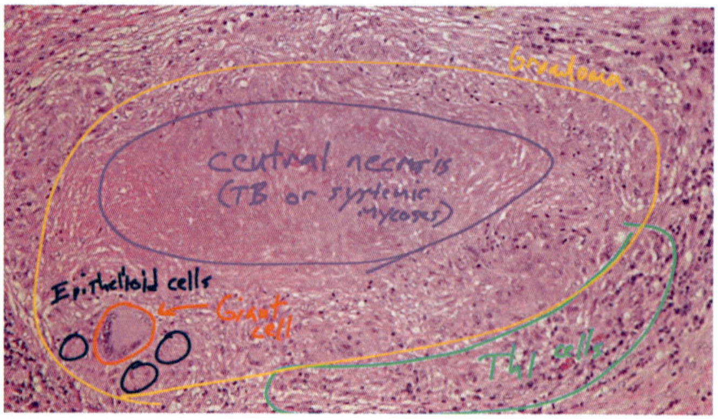

XI. Granulomas

A. Maintenance

1. Epithelioid cells (formerly macrophages) secrete TNF → granuloma remains intact

2. TNF inhibitors → granuloma breakdown → possible disease dissemination (eg, disseminated TB)

REVIEW QUESTIONS ?

1. Within tissue experiencing chronic inflammation, a macrophage restimulates a Th1 cell. During this interaction, the macrophage utilizes what surface proteins?

- **Correct answer: B7 (CD80/86), MHC II, CD40**
  - **B7 interacts with T cell CD28**
  - **MHC II interacts with T cell CD4**
  - **CD40 interacts with T cell CD40L**

Section VIII.1 - Cytokines from Macrophages and Dendritic Cells

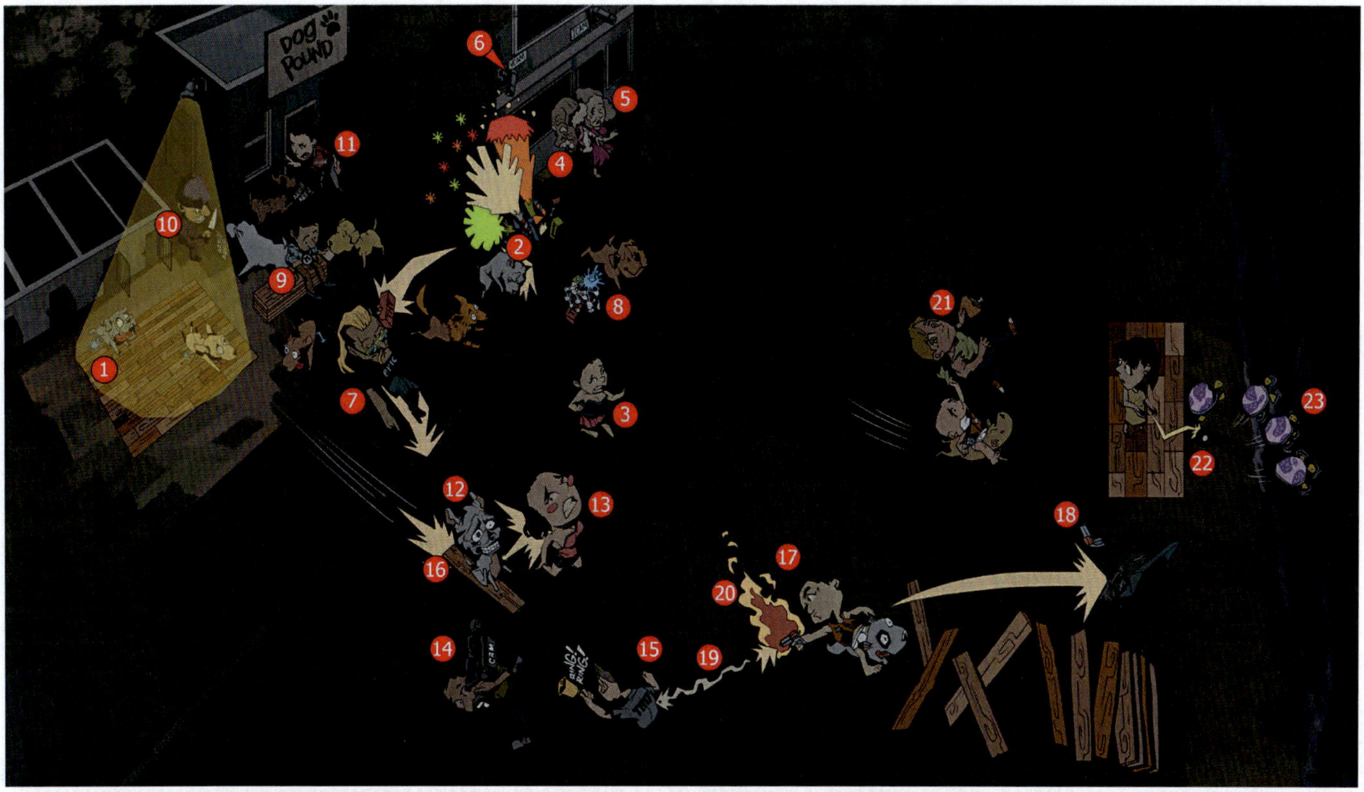

1. ______________________
2. ______________________
3. ______________________
4. ______________________
5. ______________________
6. ______________________
7. ______________________
8. ______________________
9. ______________________
10. ______________________
11. ______________________
12. ______________________
13. ______________________
14. ______________________
15. ______________________
16. ______________________
17. ______________________
18. ______________________
19. ______________________
20. ______________________
21. ______________________
22. ______________________
23. ______________________

Section IX - NK Cells and Cytotoxic T Cells

I. Cytotoxic T-cells (CD8+ T-cells)

A. Recognizes what to kill via MHC I

1. Abnormal cells present foreign antigens on MHC I → MHC I binds to CD8+ (Tc) → cell targeted for destruction
2. Foreign antigens can include particles from neoplastic cells, donor graft cells, or pathogens

B. Tc cell kills infected cell in one of two ways:

1. Releases perforins (creates pores) and granzymes → apoptosis
2. FasL binds to Fas on infected cell → apoptosis

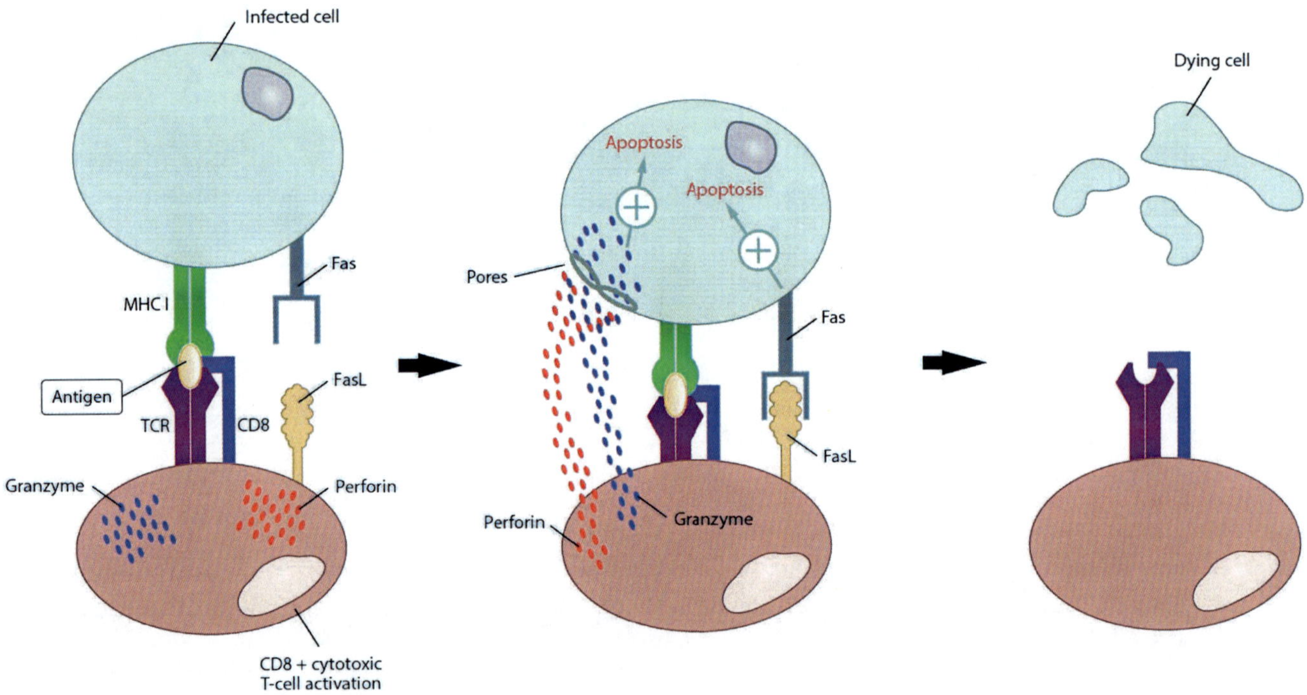

Figure 8.1.36 - Pathogen killing by Tc cells

II. Natural Killer (NK) Cells

A. Recognizes what to kill in multiple ways

1. Lack of MHC I
2. Presence of foreign surface proteins or carbohydrates
3. Antibody-dependent cell-mediated cytotoxicity (ADCC)

B. Kills infected cells in one of two ways

1. Releases perforins (creates pores) and granzymes → apoptosis
2. FasL on NK cell binds to Fas → apoptosis

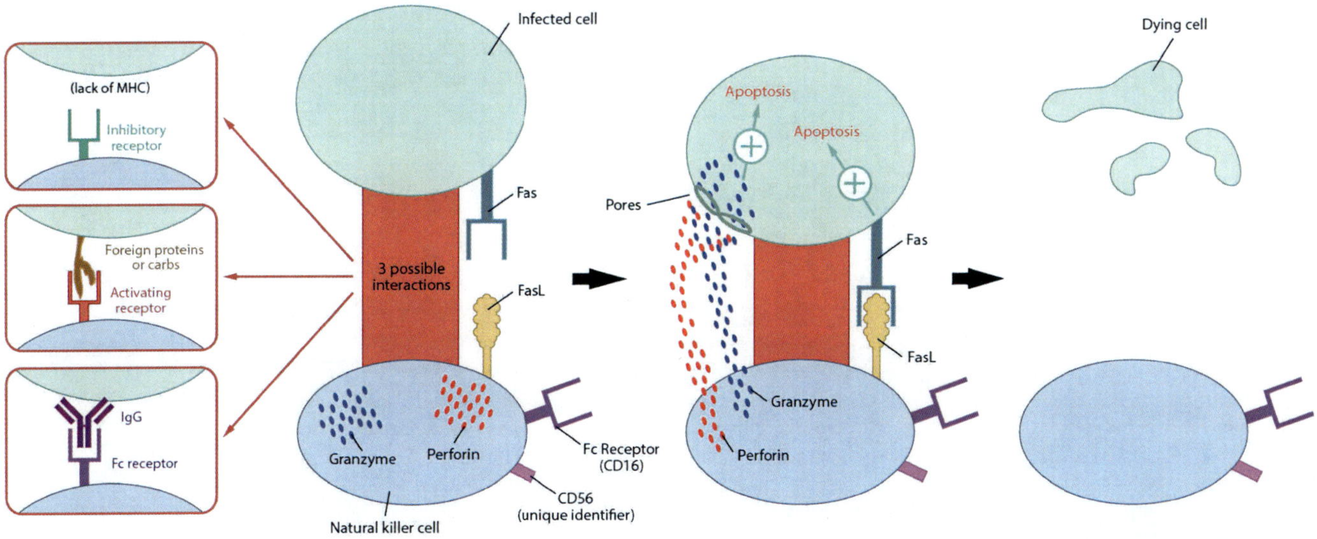

Figure 8.1.37 - Pathogen killing by natural killer cells

C. Stimulated by IFN-α, IFN-β, IL-2 and IL-12

D. Secreted cytokines

1. IFN-γ
2. IL-2

E. Surface proteins

1. CD56 (unique identifier)
2. FasL (binds to Fas)
3. CD16 (aka, Fc receptor) (binds to IgG)

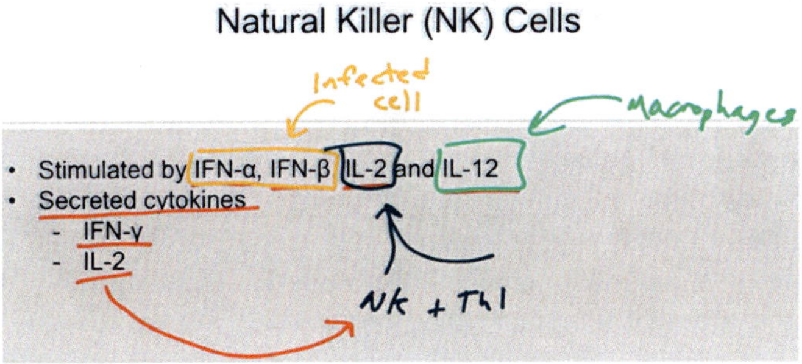

REVIEW QUESTIONS

1. After being activated by a dendritic cell, a cytotoxic T cell travels through the blood and enters the site of inflammation. The Tc cell encounters a host cell infected with a virus and induces apoptosis of that host cell. In what ways can the Tc cell can induce apoptosis?

- **Correct answer: cytotoxic T cells can induce apoptosis of infected cells in two ways:**
  - **Connection of the Fas protein to the Fas ligand**
  - **Through the release of perforins and granzymes**
- **Note: these methods are the same way in which NK cells can induce apoptosis**

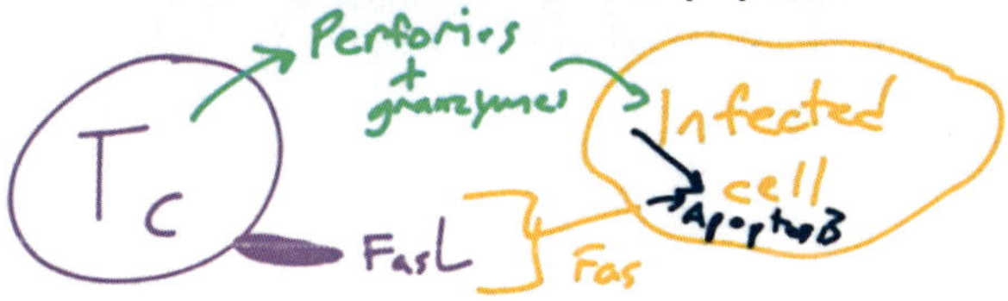

Section X - Positive and Negative Selection

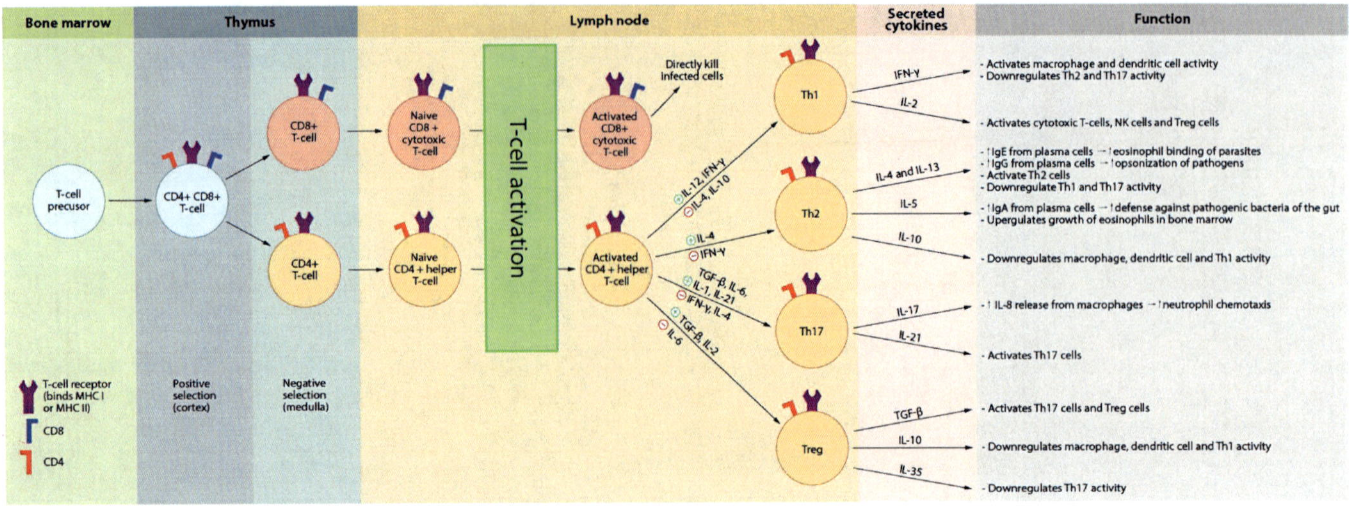

Figure 8.1.24 - T-cell differentiation and maturation

I. Positive Selection
   A. Occurs in the thymic cortex
   B. Selection for T cells that bind to self-MHC
   C. Thymic epithelial cells express self-MHC
   D. If T cells are unable to adequately bind → apoptosis
   E. If T cells successfully bind → negative selection
   F. After positive selection T cells will express either CD4 or CD8

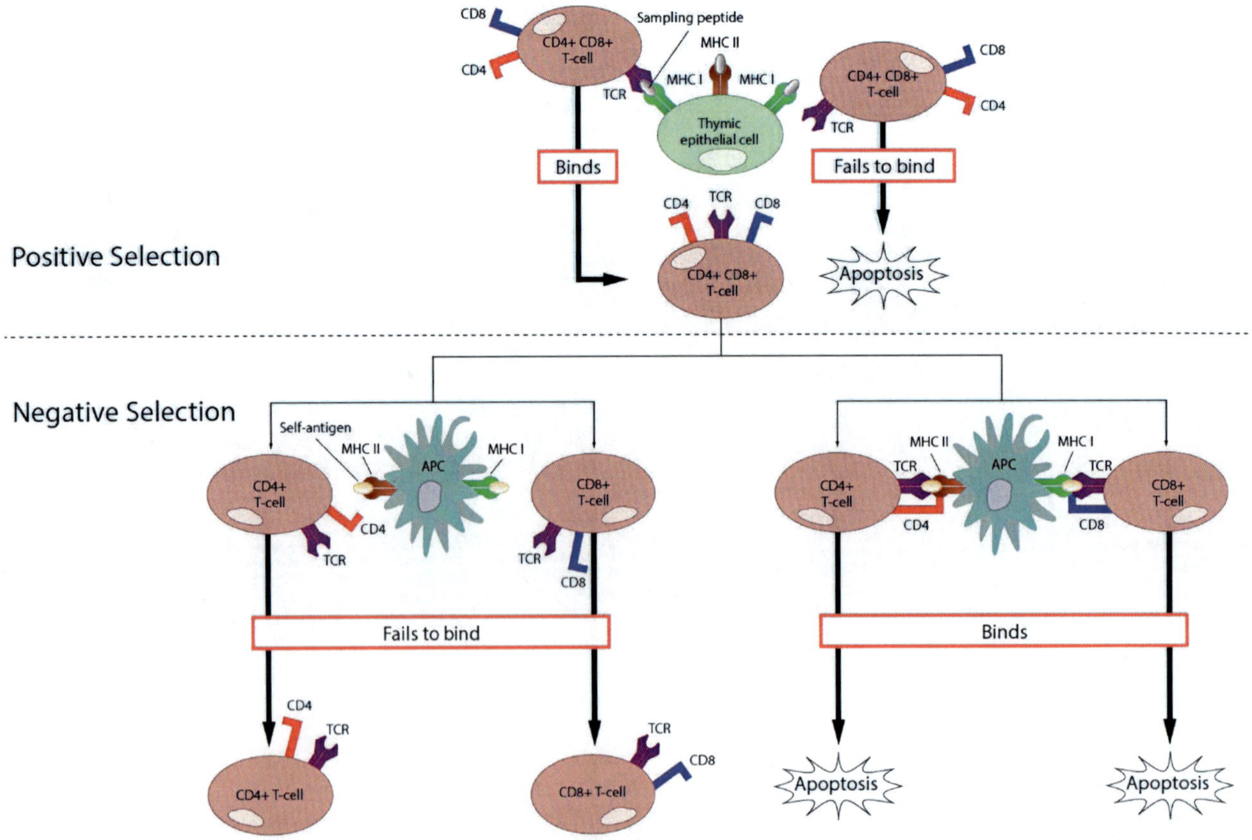

Figure 8.1.38 - Positive and negative selection

II. Negative Selection

   A. Occurs in thymic medulla

   B. Selection against T cells that bind to self antigens with high affinity

   C. Apoptosis or Treg development

III. AIRE

   A. Autoimmune regulator (AIRE) gene

   B. Responsible for intrathymic expression of self antigens

   C. Mutations → impaired negative selection

   D. Results in autoimmune endocrine diseases (eg, autoimmune polyendocrinopathy Candidiasis ectodermal dystrophy [APECED])

      1. Recurrent candida infections

      2. Hypoparathyroidism

      3. Adrenal failure

REVIEW QUESTIONS ?

1. A 37-year-old woman with a history of rheumatoid arthritis presents to her physician for follow-up care. She has several questions about how autoimmune disorders develop in relation to T-cell development. The physician informs her that her T-cells likely recognize self-antigens due to derangement of which T-cell developmental process?

   - **This patient has rheumatoid arthritis due to T-cells that likely recognize self-antigens.**
   - **Recall that these T-cells are normally destroyed during negative selection so derangement of negative selection is the correct answer.**
   - **In other words, if negative selection is messed up - patients can end up with autoimmune disorders because T-cells will mount an immune response against self-antigens.**

Section XI - T-cell Activation and Subtypes

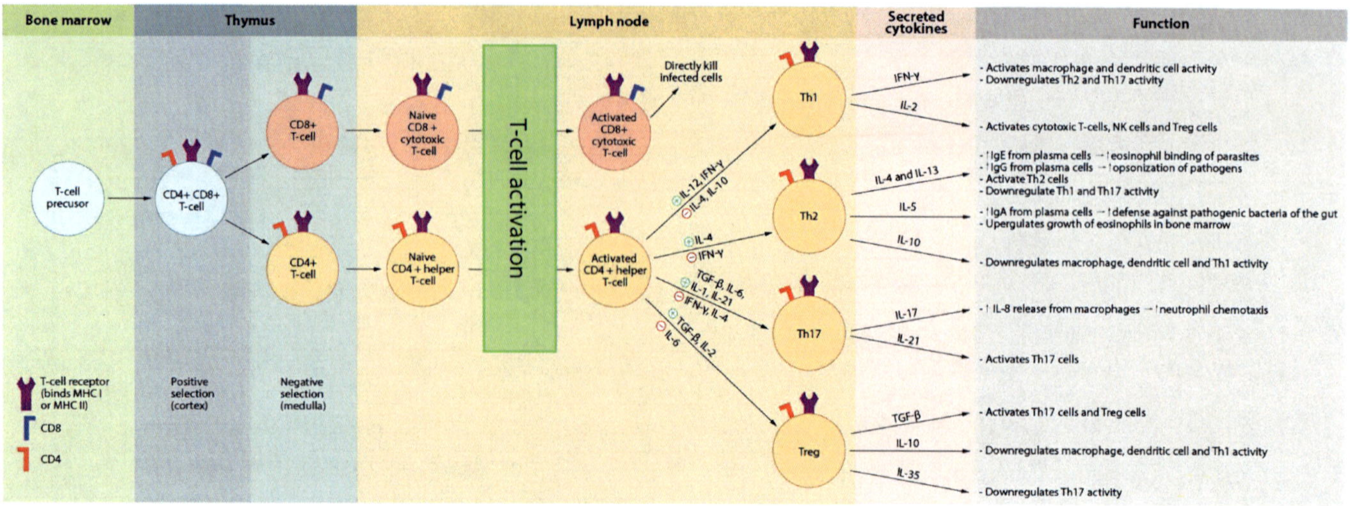

Figure 8.1.24 - T-cell differentiation and maturation

I. T-cell Activation

A. Signal 1

1. Antigen is presented on MHC I or MHC II
2. TCR binds as well as either CD4 or CD8

B. Signal 2

1. B7 protein (CD80/86) on dendritic cell and CD28 on naive T cell cause proliferation and mobilization of T-cell

C. Anergy - inability to respond to antigens

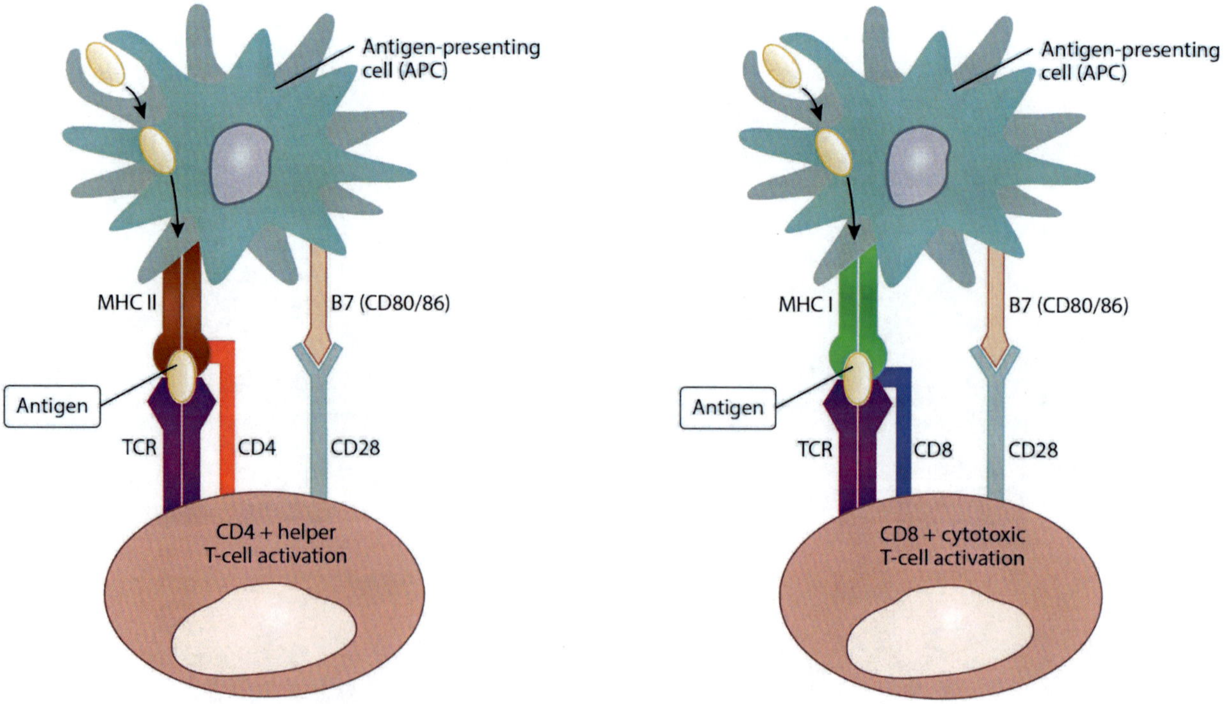

Figure 8.1.39 - T-cell activation

II. T-cell Subsets

A. Helper T cells can further subdivide based on cytokine stimulation

B. Dendritic cells facilitate this process

III. IPEX Syndrome

A. FOXP3 mutation → ↓Treg cells → autoimmunity

B. Immune dysregulation

C. Polyendocrinopathy

D. Enteropathy

E. X-linked (more common in males)

F. Other features include nail dystrophy, dermatitis, and diabetes

REVIEW QUESTIONS ?

1. After dendritic cells travel to the lymph nodes, they present foreign antigens on MHC class II molecules to T helper cells. The T-cell receptor along with CD4 are important in recognizing the foreign antigen. However, the T-cell cannot be activated unless it receives a co-stimulatory signal through which interaction?

- **The correct answer is B7 and CD28.**
- **This is describing MHC II presentation and T helper cell activation.**
- **The interaction between B7 and CD28 act as a co-stimulatory signal to activate T-helper cells.**

Section XI.1 - Cytokines from Th1 and NK Cells

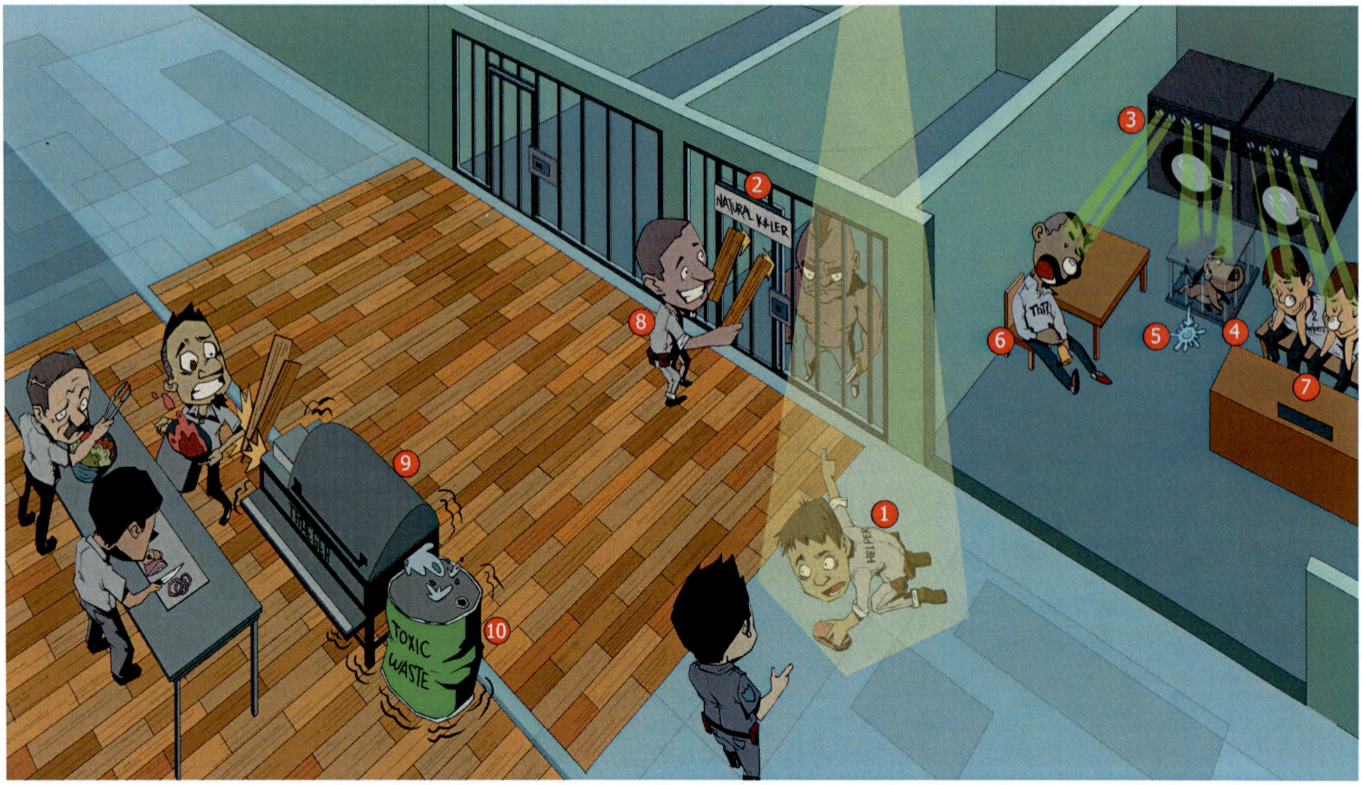

1. ______________________

2. ______________________

3. ______________________

4. ______________________

5. ______________________

6. ______________________

7. ______________________

8. ______________________

9. ______________________

10. ______________________

Section XI.2 - Cytokines from Th2 Cells

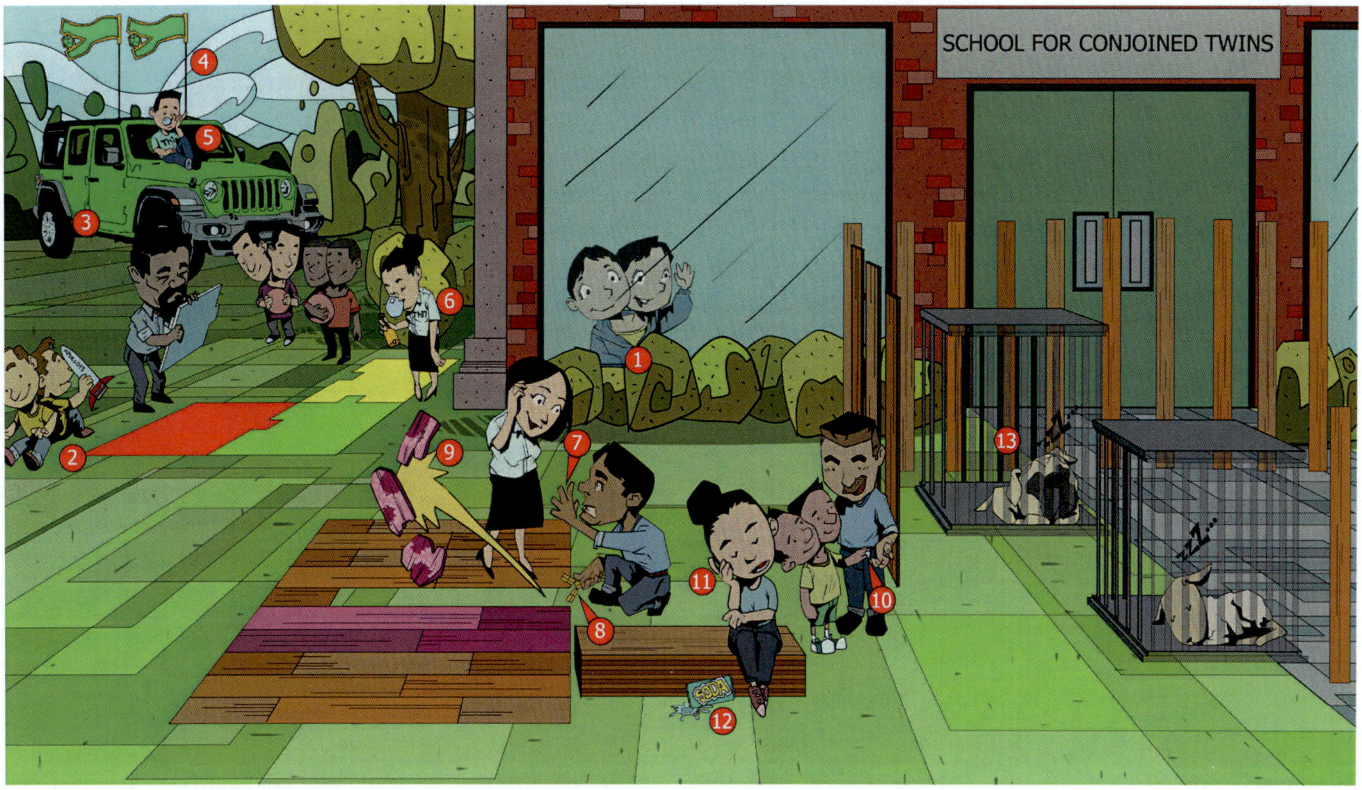

1. ______________________________
2. ______________________________
3. ______________________________
4. ______________________________
5. ______________________________
6. ______________________________
7. ______________________________
8. ______________________________
9. ______________________________
10. ______________________________
11. ______________________________
12. ______________________________
13. ______________________________

Section XI.3 - Cytokines from Th17 Cells

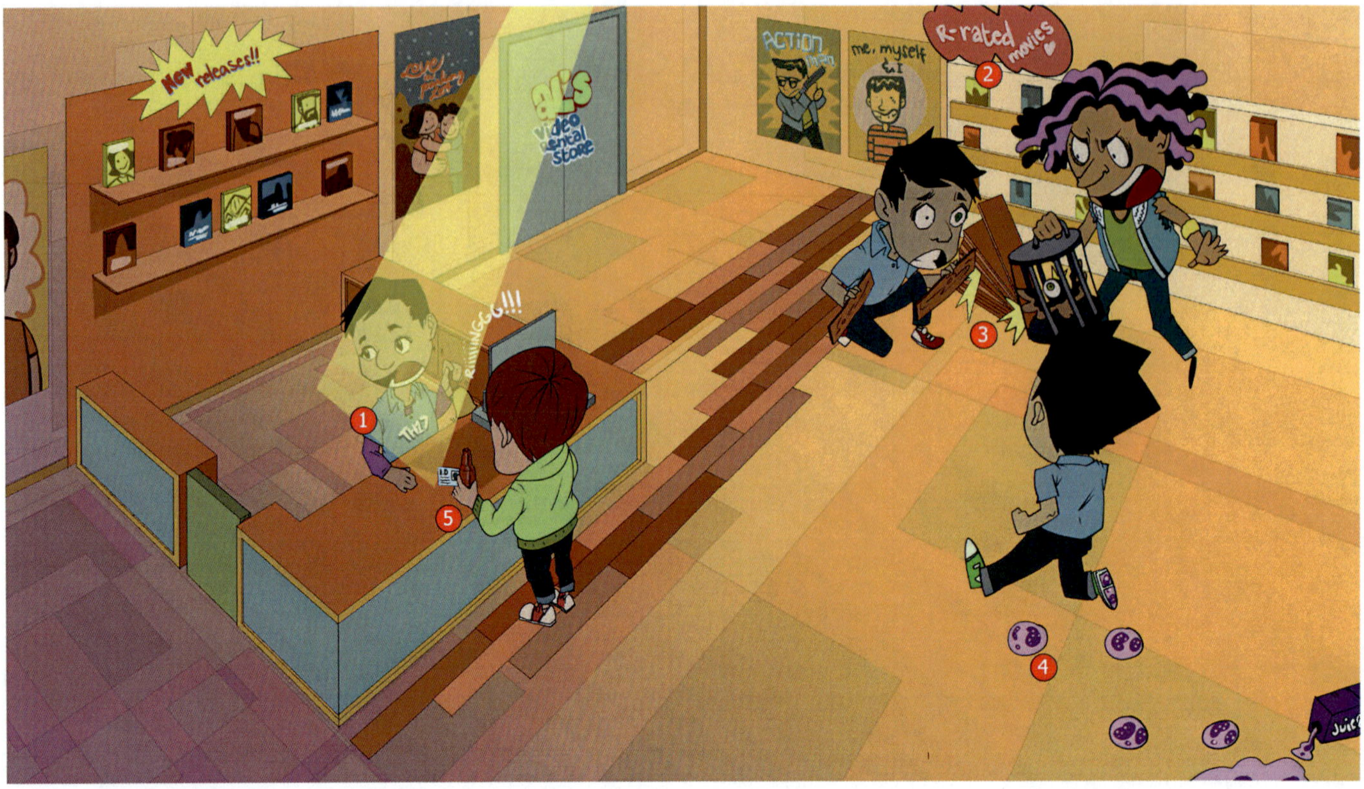

1. ______________________

2. ______________________

3. ______________________

4. ______________________

5. ______________________

Section XI.4 - Cytokines from Treg Cells

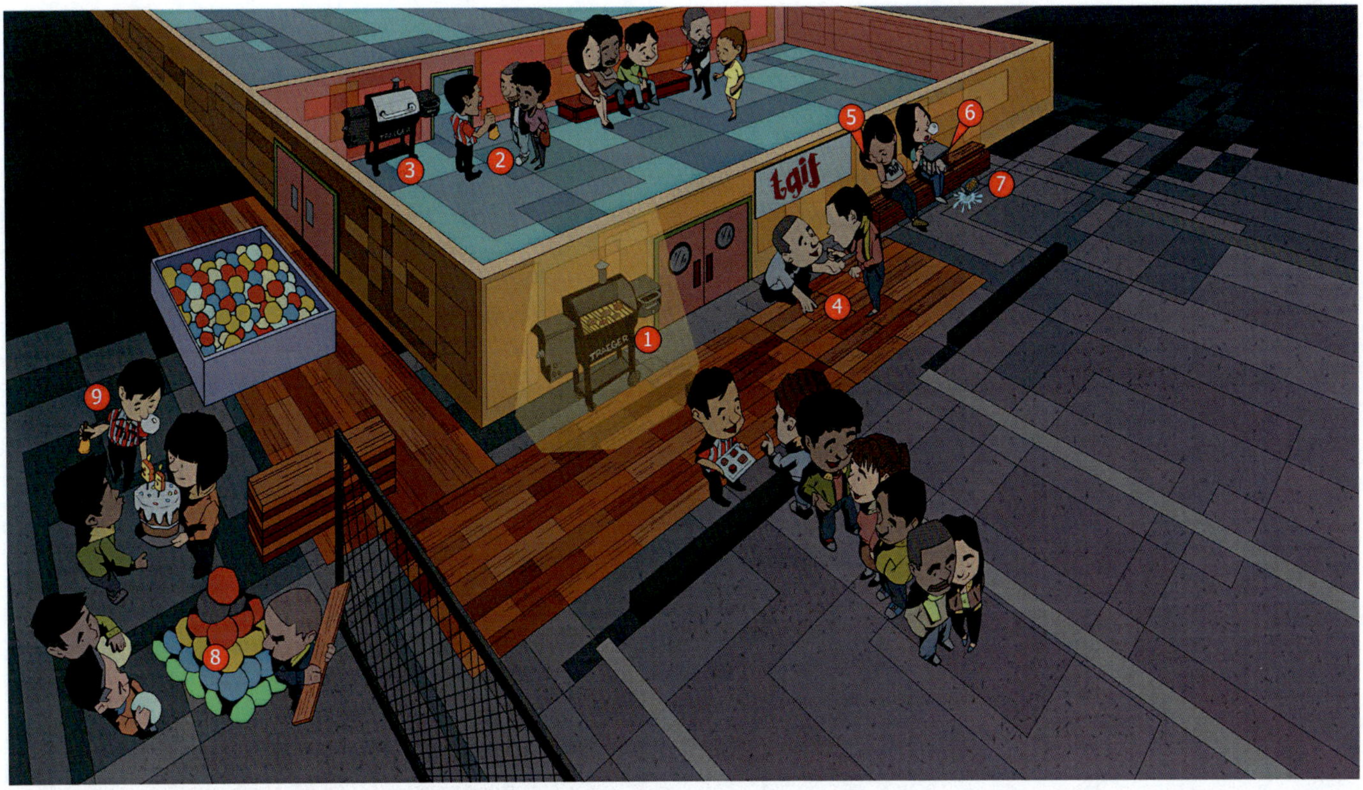

1. ______________________
2. ______________________
3. ______________________
4. ______________________
5. ______________________
6. ______________________
7. ______________________
8. ______________________
9. ______________________

Section XII - Antibodies

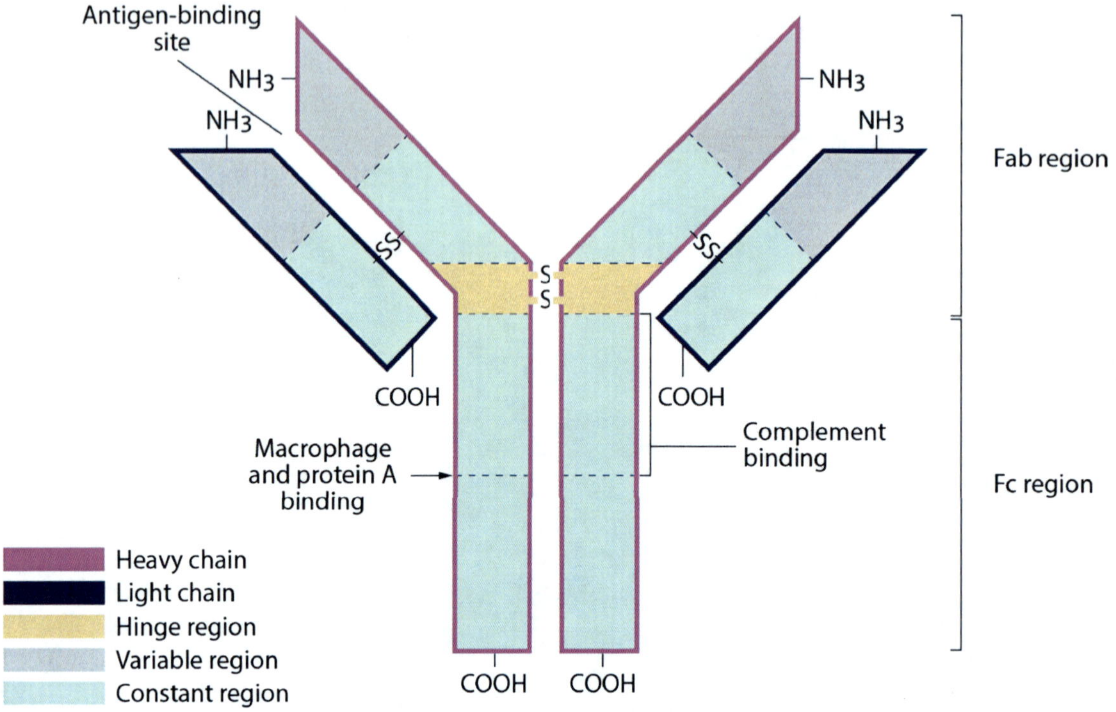

Figure 8.1.40 - Antibody structure

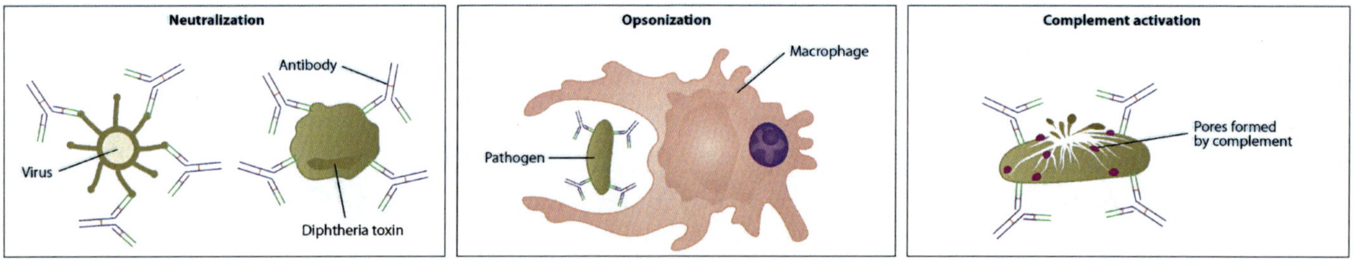

Figure 8.1.41 - Antibody function

<table>
<tr><th>Class</th><th>Complex</th><th>Description</th></tr>
<tr><td>IgM</td><td>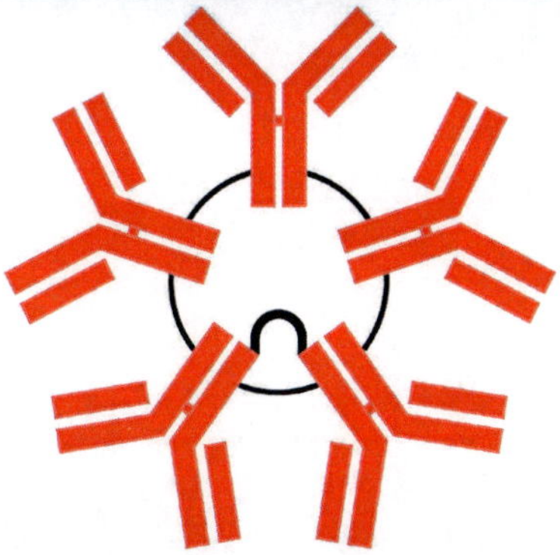</td><td>- First isotype expressed along with IgD
- Pentamer when secreted
- Monomer on B-cell surface
- Binds antigens and fixes complement
- Poor opsonization</td></tr>
<tr><td>IgD</td><td rowspan="3">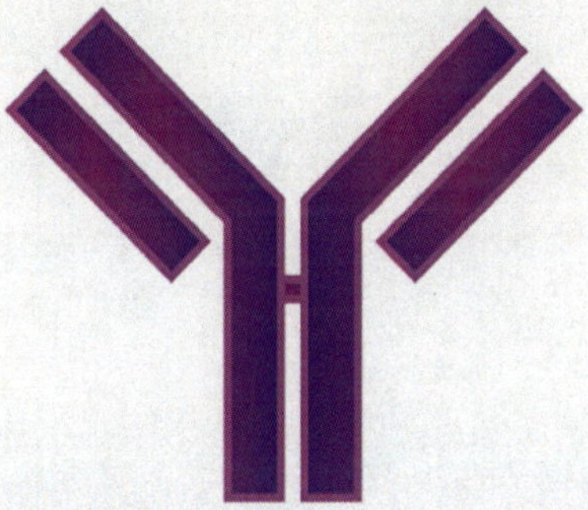</td><td>- Unknown function
- First isotype expressed along with IgM</td></tr>
<tr><td>IgG</td><td>- Most abundant isotype in serum
- Neutralization
- Opsonization
- Complement fixing
- Crosses placenta</td></tr>
<tr><td>IgE</td><td>- Binds basophils and mast cells
- Type I hypersensitivity
- Defense against parasites by activating eosinophils
- Least abundant isotype in serum</td></tr>
<tr><td>IgA</td><td>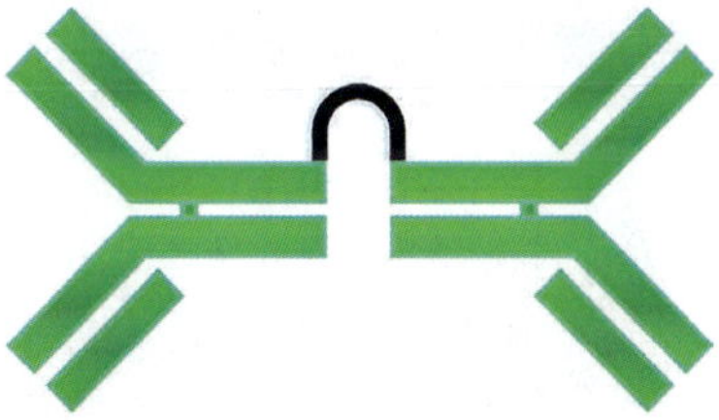</td><td>- Coats pathogens and prevents attachment to mucous membranes
- Most abundant isotype produced but low concentration in serum
- In breast milk and other secretions
- Does not fix complement
- Produced by Peyer's patches in GI tract
- Monomer in serum and dimer when secreted in tissue
- Crosses epithelial cells by transcytosis → becomes protected from luminal proteases by secretory component</td></tr>
</table>

Table 8.1.5 - Antibody isotypes and descriptions

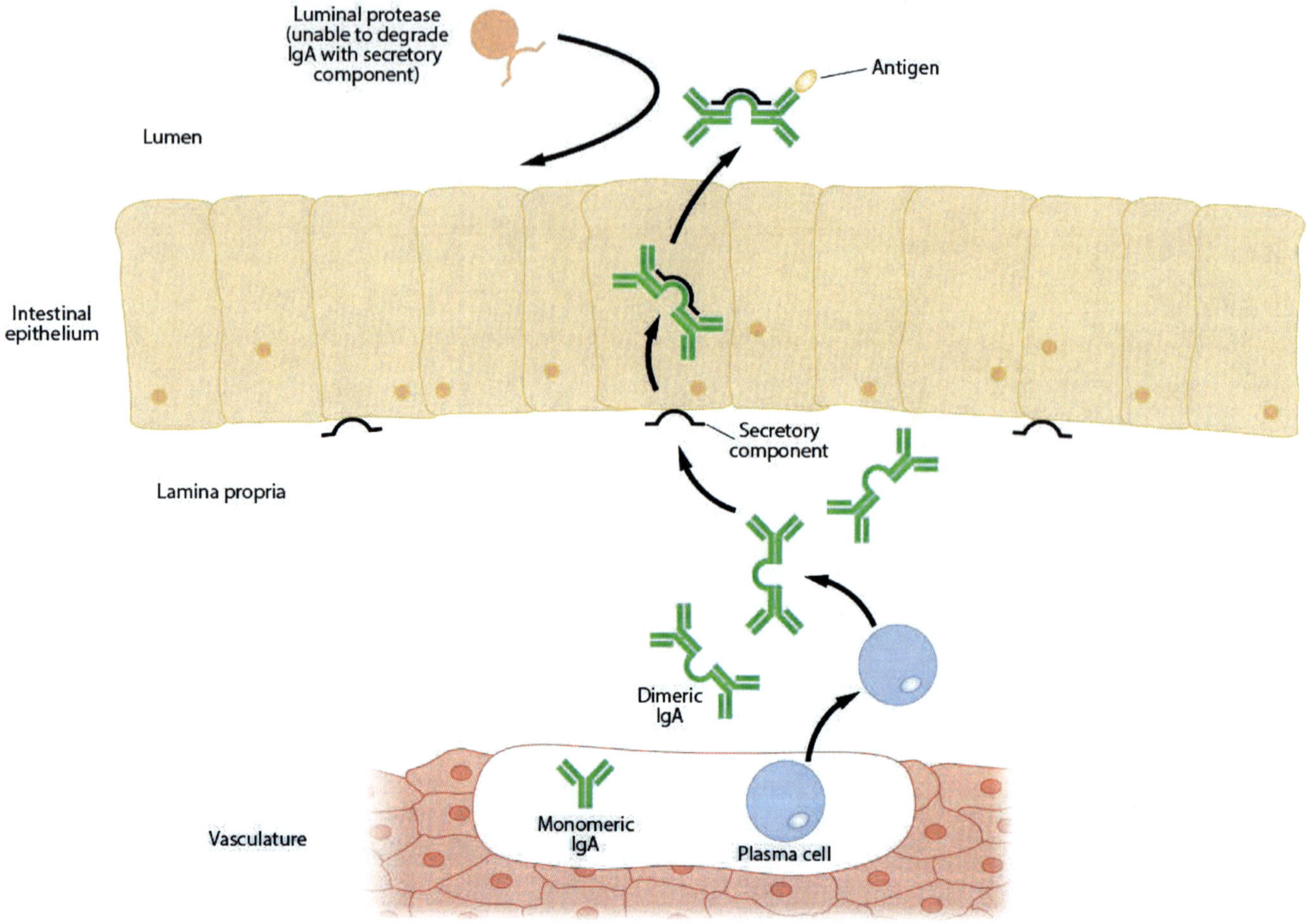

Figure 8.1.42 - IgA secretion

REVIEW QUESTIONS

1. A newborn boy develops jaundice shortly after delivery. The mother is an immigrant from Asia with little prenatal care. She has several other children all with unknown blood types. Laboratory analysis of the newborn's blood reveals maternal antibodies bound to red blood cells. What class of antibody is most likely present on the red blood cells?

- **The answer to the question is IgG.**
- **The question is describing hemolytic disease of the newborn.**
- **The mother has had little prenatal care and has several other children with unknown blood types.**
- **This is concerning for the potential exposure to Rh antigens on red blood cells from previous deliveries.**
- **Exposure to these antigens during pregnancy or delivery can cause the mother to mount an immune response.**
- **When this happens the mother can develop anti Rh IgG antibodies which can then cross the placenta and harm the developing fetus in a subsequent pregnancy.**
- **This is exactly what is being described in the question stem.**
- **Only IgG can cross the placenta.**

Section XIII - B-cells

I. B-cells

A. Derived from multipotential hematopoietic stem cells

B. Cell markers include CD19, CD20, and CD21

C. Epstein-Barr virus (EBV) uses CD21 to infiltrate B-cells

II. Overview

A. VDJ recombination (B-cell receptor development)

B. Activation (proliferation)

C. Maturation

1. Somatic hypermutation

2. Class switching

3. Differentiation

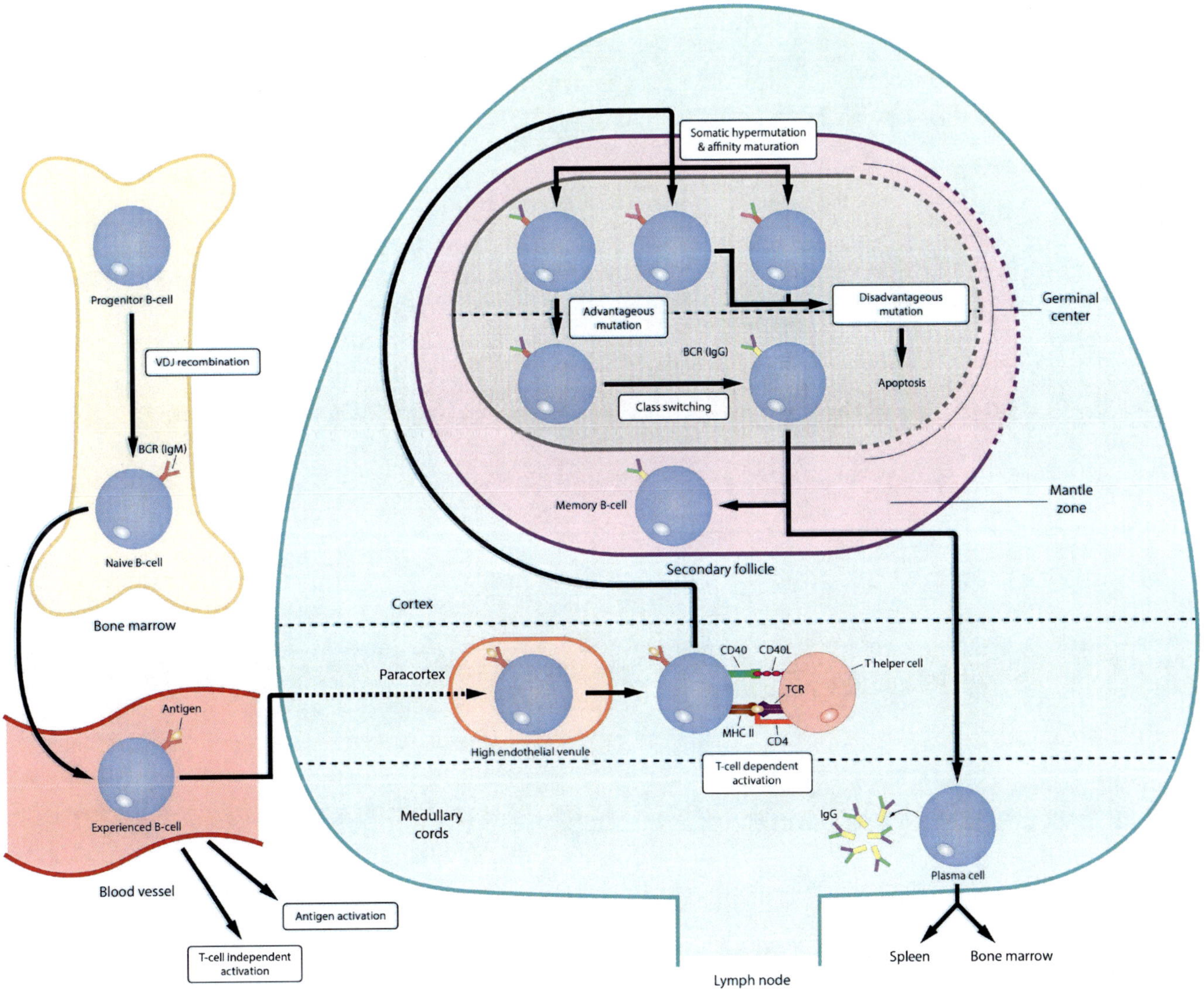

Figure 8.1.43 - B-cell development

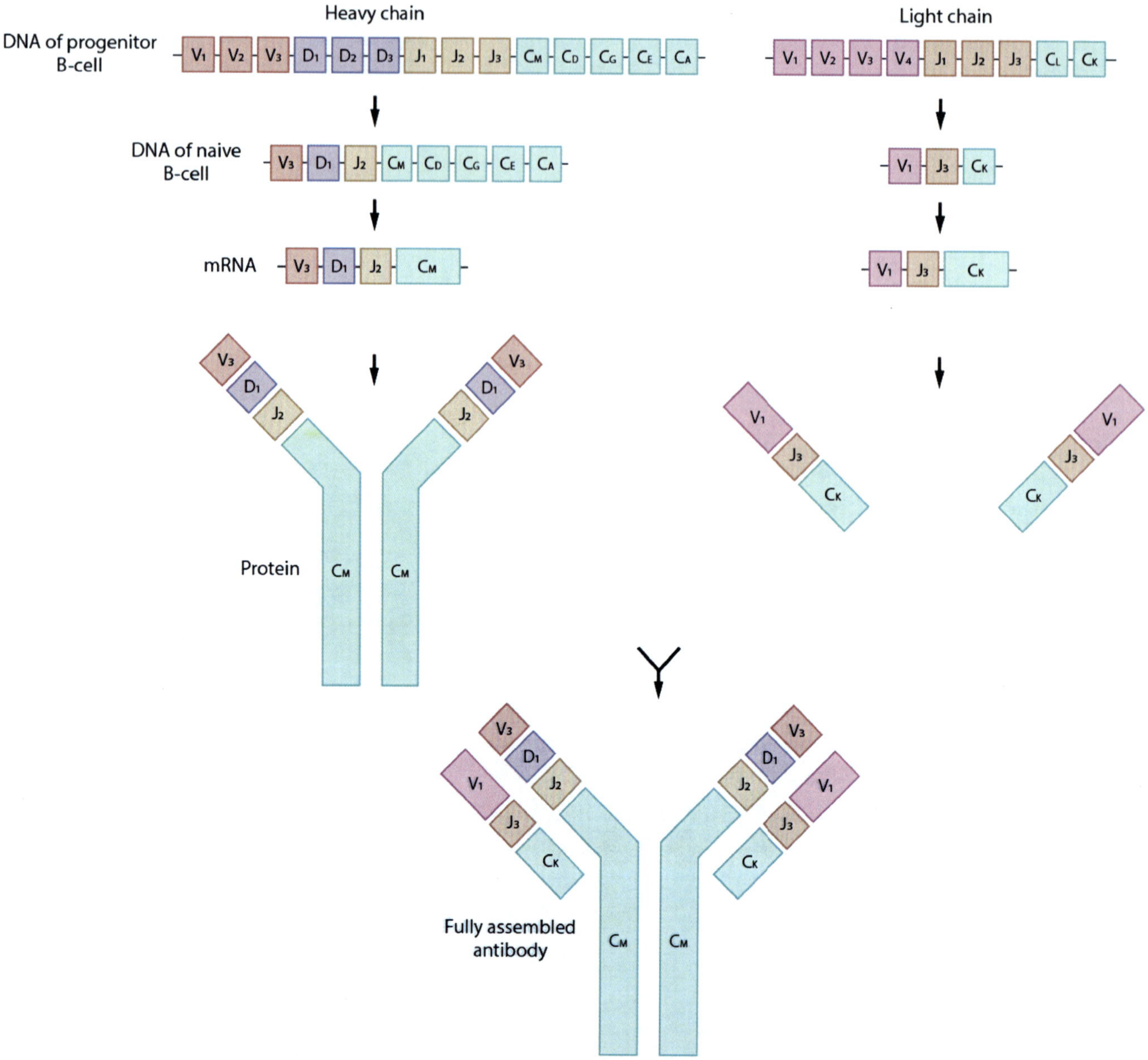

Figure 8.1.44 - VDJ recombination

III. VDJ Recombination

A. The process by which the B-cell develops antibody diversity including generation of a unique B-cell receptor

B. Variable (V), diversity (D), and joining (J) DNA segments are randomly removed during B-cell development

C. The VDJ and C regions are transcribed into mRNA, translated into protein, and combined with proteins from the light chain → fully assembled antibody

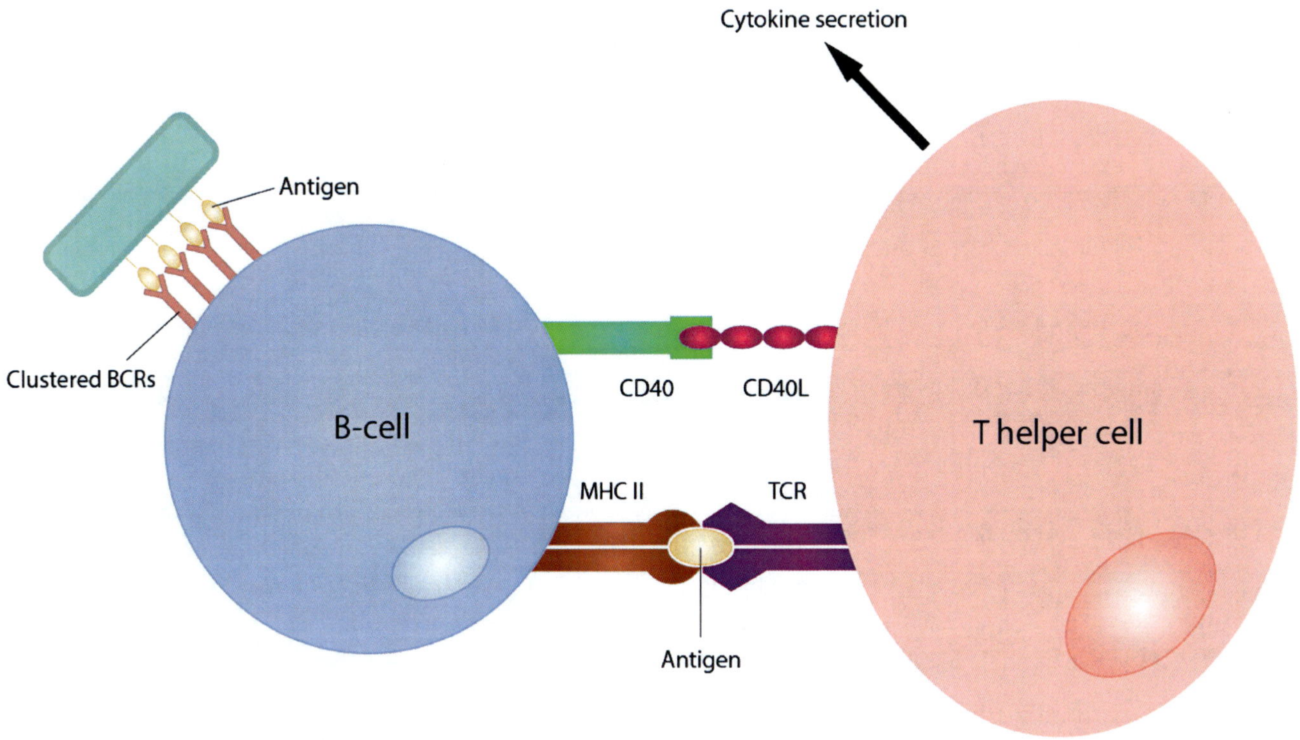

Figure 8.1.45 - T-cell dependent activation of B-cells

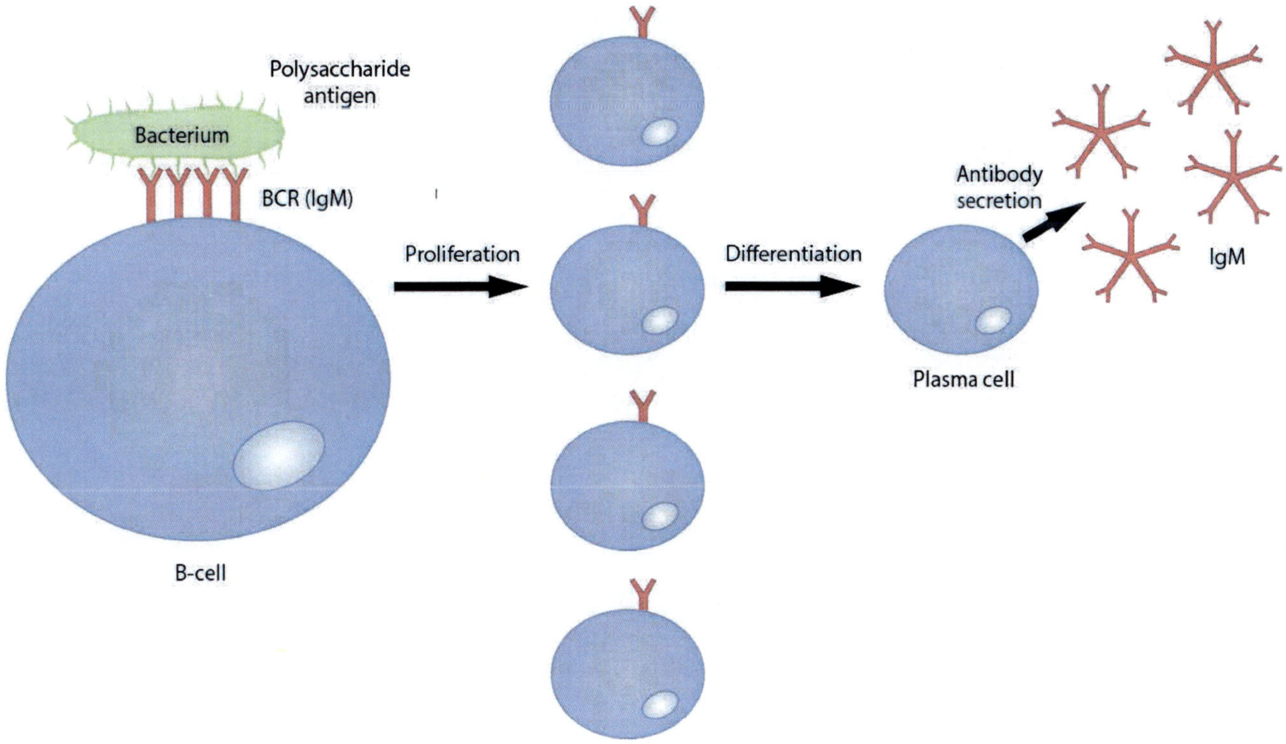

Figure 8.1.46 - T-cell independent activation of B-cells

IV. Activation

A. T-cell dependent activation

1. B-cell travels to the lymph node
2. Activated by T helper cell

B. T-cell independent activation

1. B-cell activated by non-protein antigens (e.g., polysaccharides)

C. Antigen activation

1. Antigen binds and clusters non B-cell receptors → BCRs become clustered → activation

V. Somatic Hypermutation & Affinity Maturation

A. Somatic hypermutation: a large number of rapid mutations that occur in the DNA responsible for producing the variable region of the BCR

B. Affinity maturation: the BCR with a greater affinity for the antigen will be allowed to mature

VI. Class Switching

A. Allows the B-cell to change the class of antibody it produces

B. Default antibody is IgM

C. Only after class switching can IgG, IgA, or IgE be produced

D. A constant segment of DNA is removed (e.g., IgM) and the remaining constant region (e.g., IgG) is then translated and combined with the same variable regions

VII. Differentiation

A. B-cells can differentiate into memory cells or plasma cells

B. Memory cells migrate to the mantle zone of the secondary follicle

C. Reexposure to the antigen immediately generates an antibody-mediated immune response via memory cells

D. Plasma cells secrete antibodies

REVIEW QUESTIONS ?

1. A 2-year-old boy with a history of recurrent pyogenic infections is found to have a defect in CD40L on T helper cells. Immunoglobulins present in the patient's serum are analyzed. Which immunoglobulin(s) will most likely be elevated and which one(s) will be decreased?

- **IgM will be elevated while IgG, IgA, and IgE will all be low.**
- **From the question we're told that CD40 ligand on T helper cells is defective.**
- **We're then asked about immunoglobulins.**
- **We talk more about this in our immunodeficiency videos, but this question is describing Hyper IgM syndrome which results in elevated levels of IgM and depressed levels of all other immunoglobulins.**
- **CD40 ligand is necessary for the B-cell to class switch.**
- **Therefore, a CD40 ligand defect will result in the patient only being able to produce IgM.**

Section XIV - Vaccinations

I. Vaccine Overview

A. The ideal vaccine maximizes immunologic memory while minimizing side effects, including infection

1. Good: forming memory B cells
2. Better: forming memory B cells and memory Th cells
3. Best: forming memory B cells, memory Th cells, and memory Tc cells

Vaccine	Description	Examples	Notes
Live (attenuated)	- Whole, live pathogen - Virulence factors have been removed - Induces a humoral response → memory Th and memory B cells - Induces a cellular response → memory Tc cells	- Adenovirus, S. typhi (oral), Polio (Sabin), Varicella, Smallpox, BCG (TB), Influenza (intranasal), Yellow fever, MMR, Rotavirus	- Pathogen can mutate and acquire a virulence factor → infection (contraindicated in immunodeficiency and pregnancy)
Killed (inactivated)	- Whole, killed pathogen - Induces a humoral response → memory Th and memory B cells	- Rabies, Influenza (IM), Polio (Salk), HAV, S. typhi (IM)	- Requires booster

Subunit	- Subunits are selected antigens from a killed pathogen
	- Recombinant DNA technology is often used to procure only the desired antigen (eg, yeast growing HBsAg)
	- Induces a humoral response
	  - Polysaccharides → T-cell independent activation of B cells → memory B cells only (and only IgM)
	  - Proteins → T-cell dependent activation of B cells → memory B cells and memory Th cells
	  - Toxoid (denatured bacterial exotoxin) → T-cell dependent activation of B cells → memory B cells and memory Th cells
	- Antigens may be combined with another substance to increase the immune response (assume nearly every vaccine has been combined)
	  - Protein conjugate → memory Th and memory B cells
	  - Adjuvant (eg, aluminum) → ↑ TLR recognition → ↑ phagocytosis → ↑ dendritic cell presentation → memory Th and memory B cells
		- Polysaccharides:
		S. pneumoniae
		H. influenzae type b
		N. meningitidis
		- Proteins:
		HBV (HBsAg)
		HPV (capsid proteins from 6, 11, 16, and 18)
		- Toxoids:
		DTaP (Diphtheria toxoid, Tetanus toxoid, and acellular Pertussis antigens)
			- Requires booster
			- Expensive

Table 8.1.6 - Vaccinations

II. Humoral vs. Cellular Immunity

A. The immune system is comprised of innate and adaptive responses

B. The adaptive immune system includes humoral and cellular responses

C. Humoral = Helper T cells (interleukins) and B cells (antibodies)

1. Memory Th cells and memory B cells are formed

D. Cellular = Cytotoxic T cells (killing infected cells)

1. Memory Tc cells are formed

III. Cross-presentation on MHC I

A. MHC I is present on all nucleated cells

B. Infected cells present antigens on MHC I → mark the cell for killing (this does not activate naive Tc cells)

C. Infected dendritic cells can present on MHC I ("cross-presentation") → Tc (CD8+) activation

1. Assumption 1: dendritic cells are infected when they activate naive Tc cells in the lymph node

2. Assumption 2: only live vaccines can infect dendritic cells and cause a cellular response (Tc cell activation)

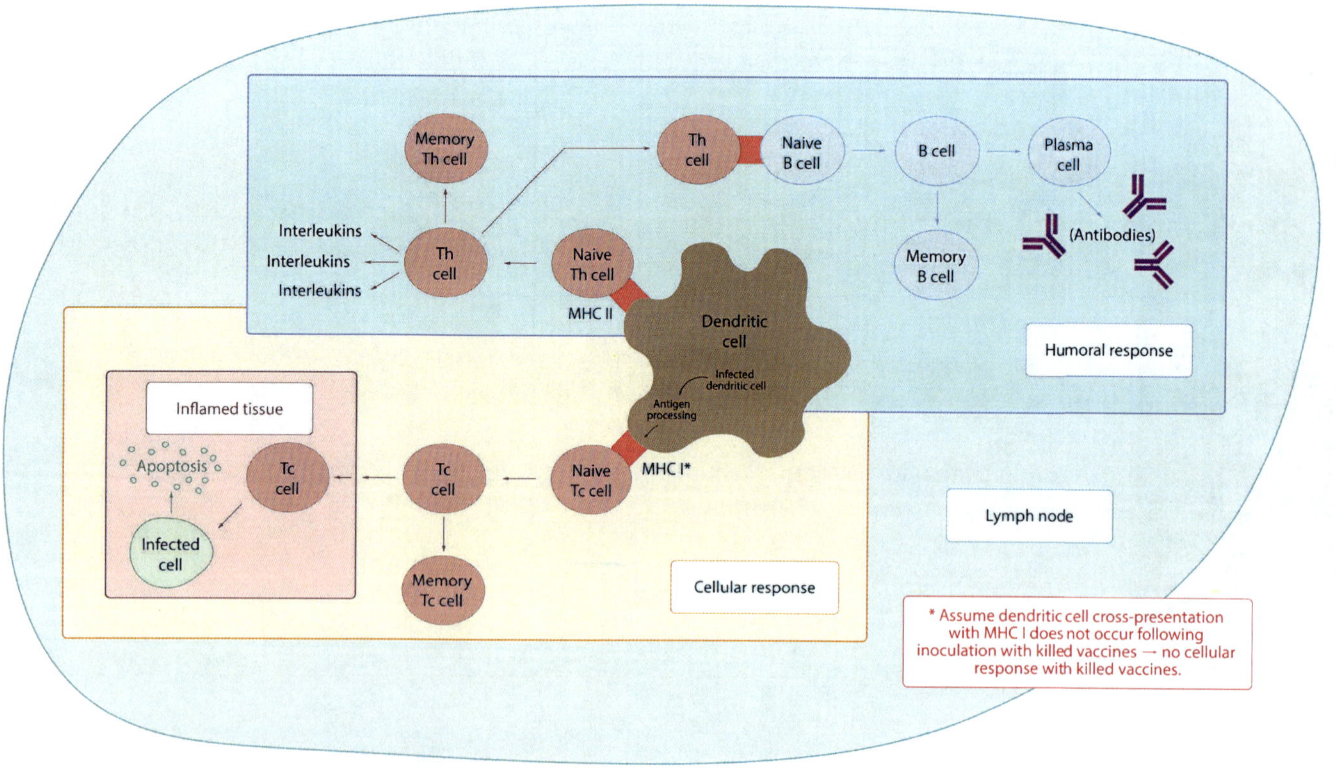

Figure 8.1.47 - Humoral and cellular immunity

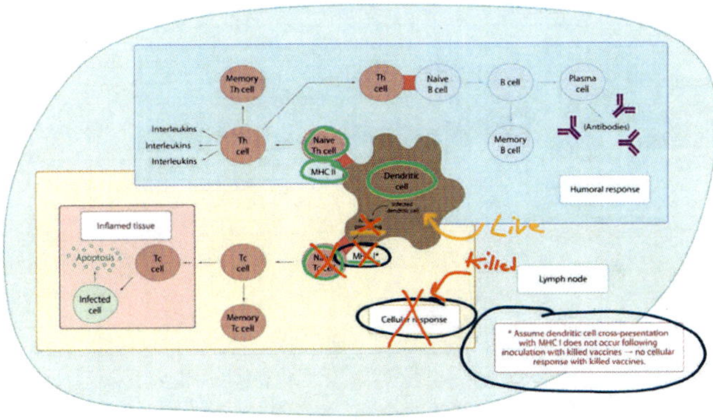

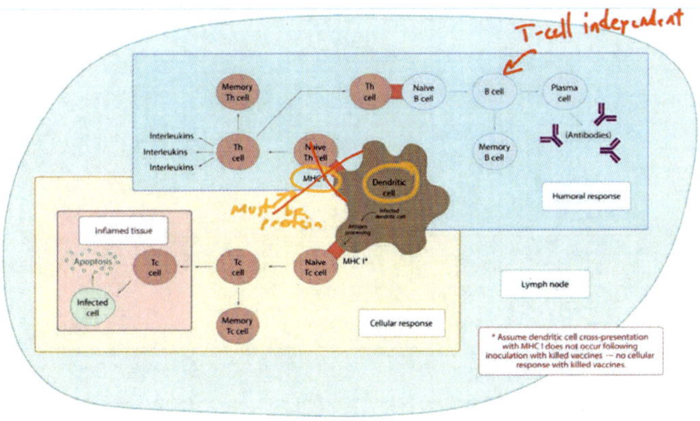

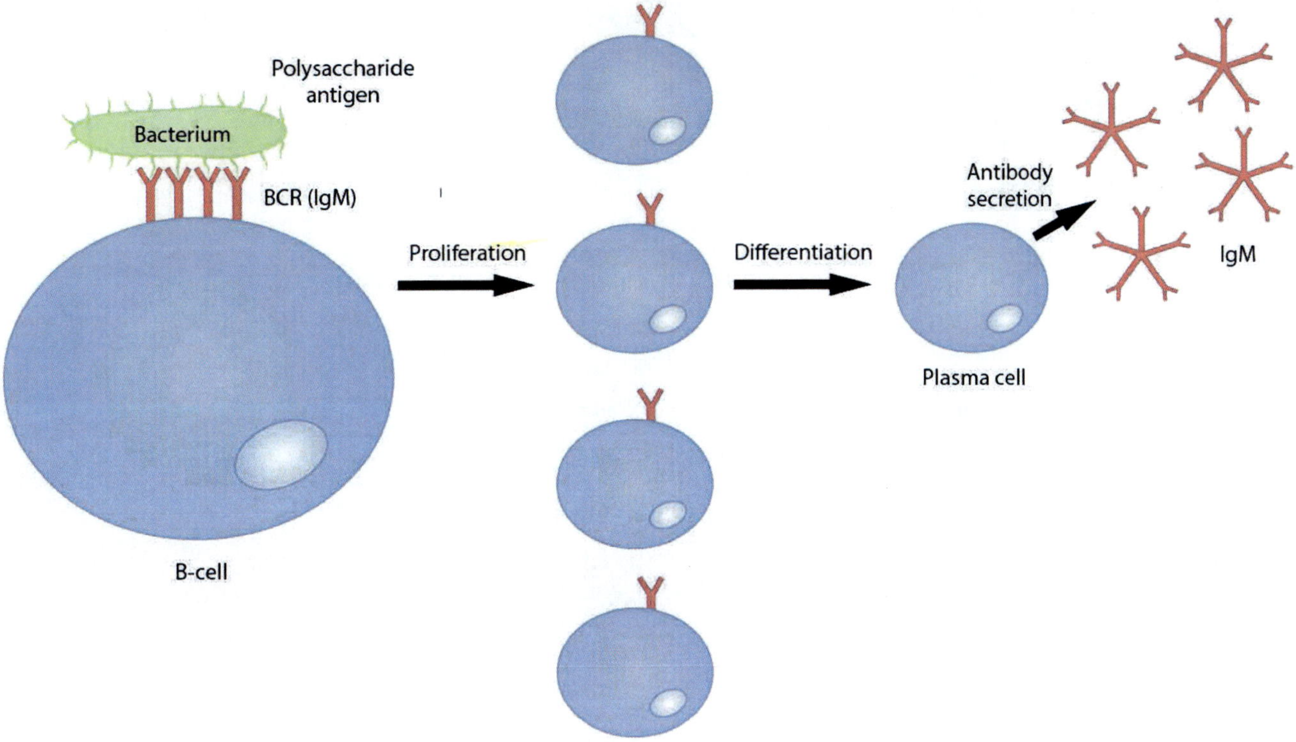

Figure 8.1.46 - T-cell independent activation of B-cells

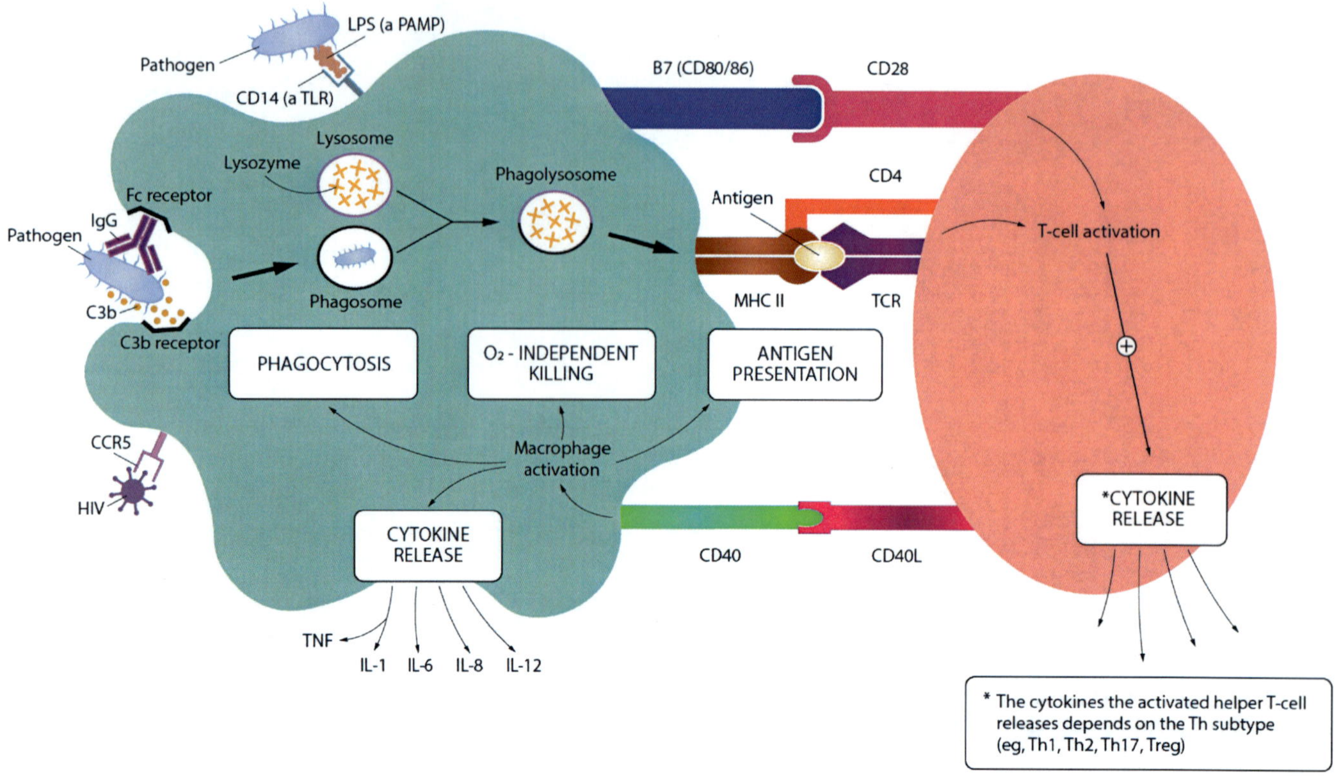

Figure 8.1.31 - Macrophage interaction with T cell

REVIEW QUESTIONS

?

1. A pharmaceutical company is attempting to create a novel vaccine that targets the polysaccharides on the capsule of E. coli. Their goal is to avoid using conjugate proteins or adjuvants in their vaccine formulation. If the vaccine works, what type of immunologic memory should be expected?

   - **Correct answer: Memory B cells**
   - **Reason through the question this way: this vaccine only targets polysaccharides → must be a subunit vaccine → subunits induce T-cell independent activation of B cells → only B cells are activated (not Tc or Th cells) → memory B cells**
   - **To form memory Th cells, the vaccine must be a whole pathogen**
   - **To form memory Tc cells, the vaccine must be a whole pathogen and be live**

Live (whole)
Killed (whole)
Subunit (polysaccharides only)

Memory B
~~memory~~ Th
~~memory~~ Tc

Section XV - Hypersensitivity Reactions

I. Hypersensitivity

A. Unintended immune response that causes disease

B. Immune system becomes "sensitized" following initial antigen exposure

C. Hypersensitivity occurs following second antigen exposure

D. Four types

Type	Description	Examples	Other
I	-Immediate (minutes): free antigens crosslink IgE on presensitized mast cells → degranulation → histamine & tryptase → anaphylaxis or atopy -Late (hours): leukotrienes and chemokines → tissue damage	- Asthma - Anaphylaxis (drug reactions, bee sting, food) -Seasonal allergies	- ELISA blood test or intradermal skin test can detect allergen-specific IgE
II	-Antibody binds to antigen on target cell → destruction, inflammation, and dysfunction -Destruction is due to opsonization → complement activation and phagocytosis or NK cell-mediated apoptosis -Inflammation is due to complement activation -Dysfunction is due to antibody-mediated blockade of cell surface receptors	- Transfusion reactions (ABO incompatibility) - Hemolytic disease of the newborn - Graves' disease	- Direct Coombs test: detects antibodies on the surface of RBCs - Indirect Coombs test: detects antibodies in the serum
III	-Antigen and antibody form immune complexes → deposition in tissues → activation of complement (causes hypocomplementemia) → inflammation (eg, neutrophil chemotaxis, mast cell degranulation) -Serum sickness: widespread deposition of immune complexes following exposure to a protein antigen from a nonhuman species (eg, infliximab) → rash, malaise, fever, and polyarthralgias days to weeks following exposure -Arthus reaction: local deposition of immune complexes (injected antigen binds to presensitized IgG resulting in immune complex formation) typically following a vaccine booster (eg, diphtheria, tetanus, HBV) → local pain, swelling, erythema	- Post-streptococcal glomerulonephritis - Infliximab (serum sickness) - Penicillin (serum sickness-like reaction)	- Serum sickness-like reactions are less severe and can be caused by infections (eg, HBV) and drugs (eg, penicillin)
IV	-T-cell mediated. Also known as delayed-type hypersensitivity (requires time due to T-cell involvement). -CD8+ cytotoxic T-cells directly kill cells -CD4+ T-cells are stimulated to release inflammatory-inducing cytokines after antigen recognition	- Contact dermatitis (eg, nickel allergy, poison ivy) - Candida antigen exposure - Purified protein derivative (PPD) test - Transplant rejection	- The only hypersensitivity reaction that is not mediated by antibodies

Table 8.1.7 - Hypersensitivity reactions

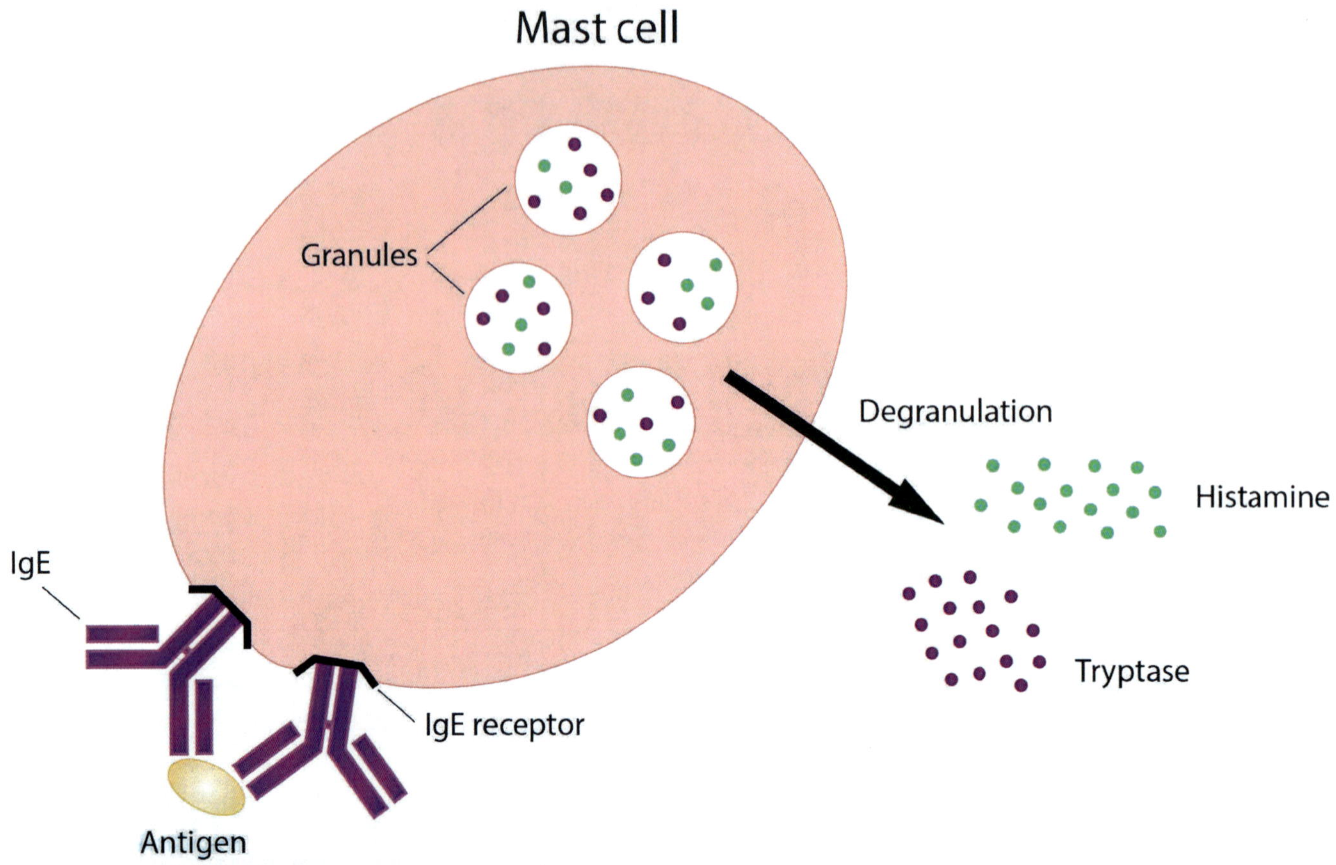

Figure 8.1.48 - Type I hypersensitivity reaction (mast cell degranulation)

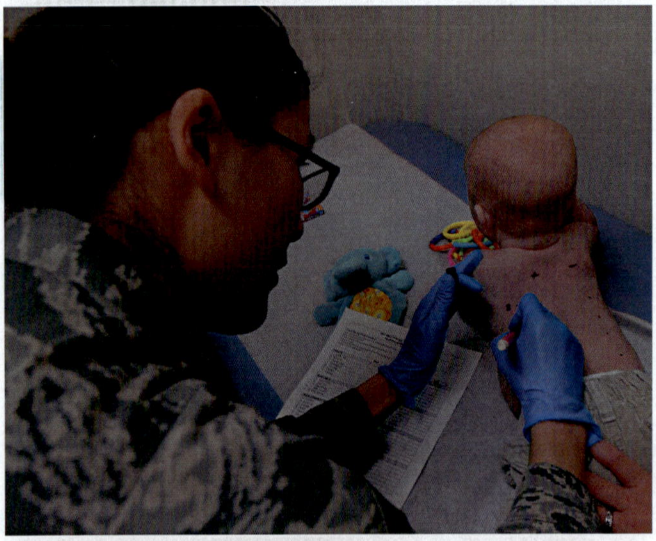

Photo Credit: Airman St Class Austin HarvillRleased (https://www.jble.af.mil/News/Photos/igphoto/2000072328/)

Figure 8.1.49 - Allergy test

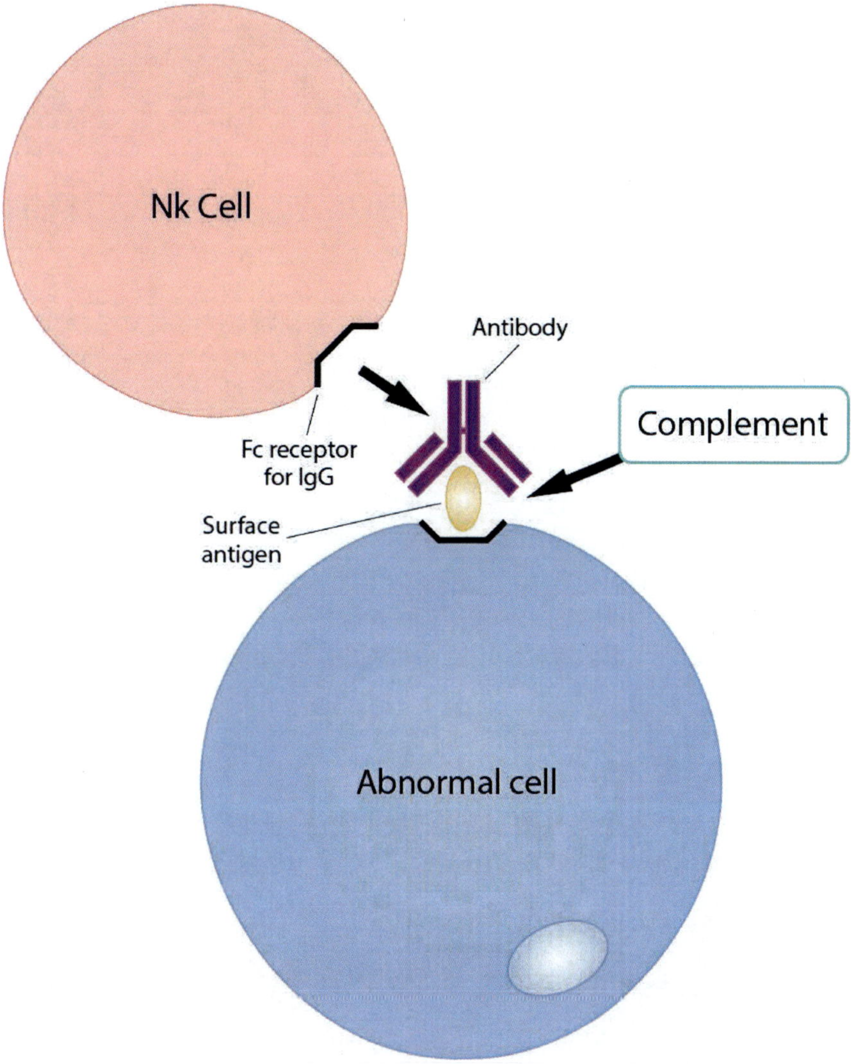

Figure 8.1.50 - Type II hypersensitivity reaction (antibody binds to target cell)

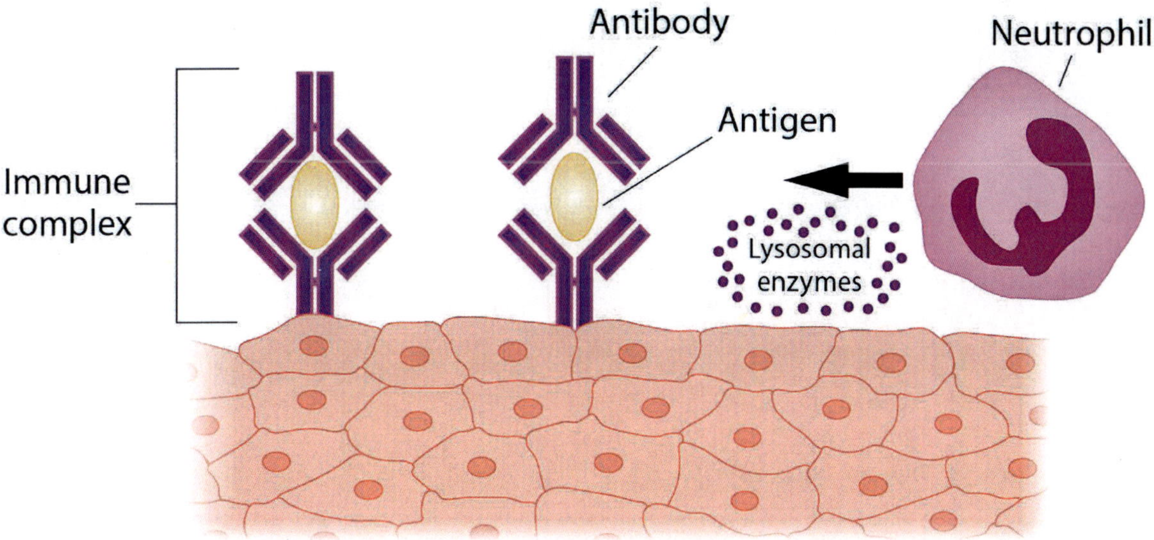

Figure 8.1.51 - Type III hypersensitivity reaction (immune complex deposition)

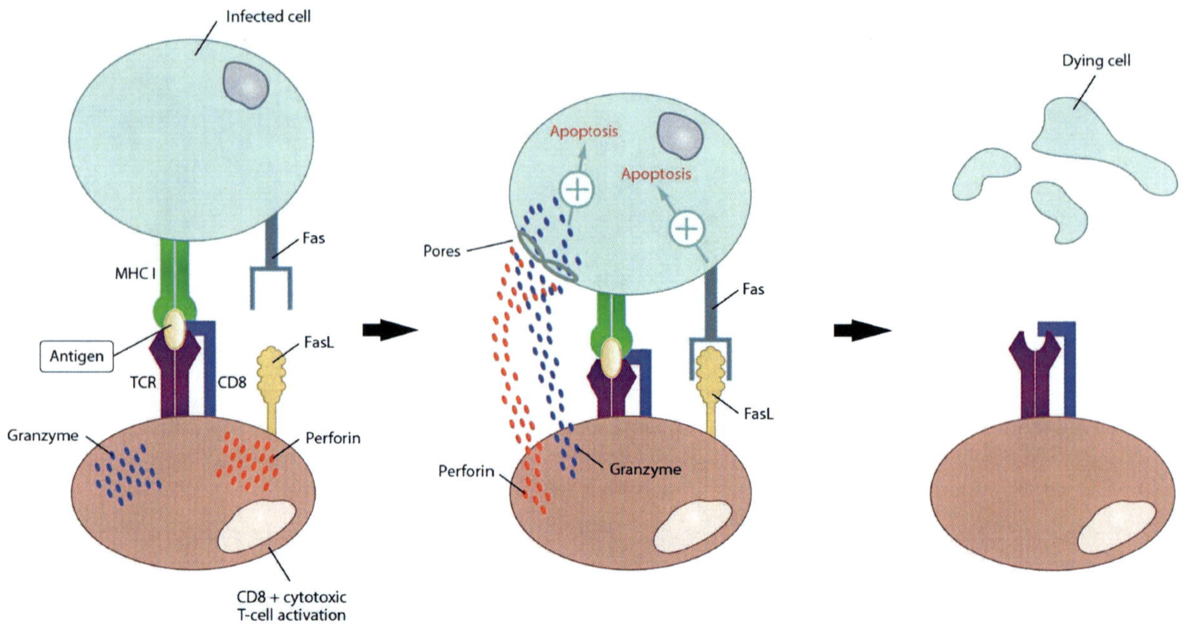

Figure 8.1.52 - Type IV hypersensitivity reaction (CD8+ T-cell mediated)

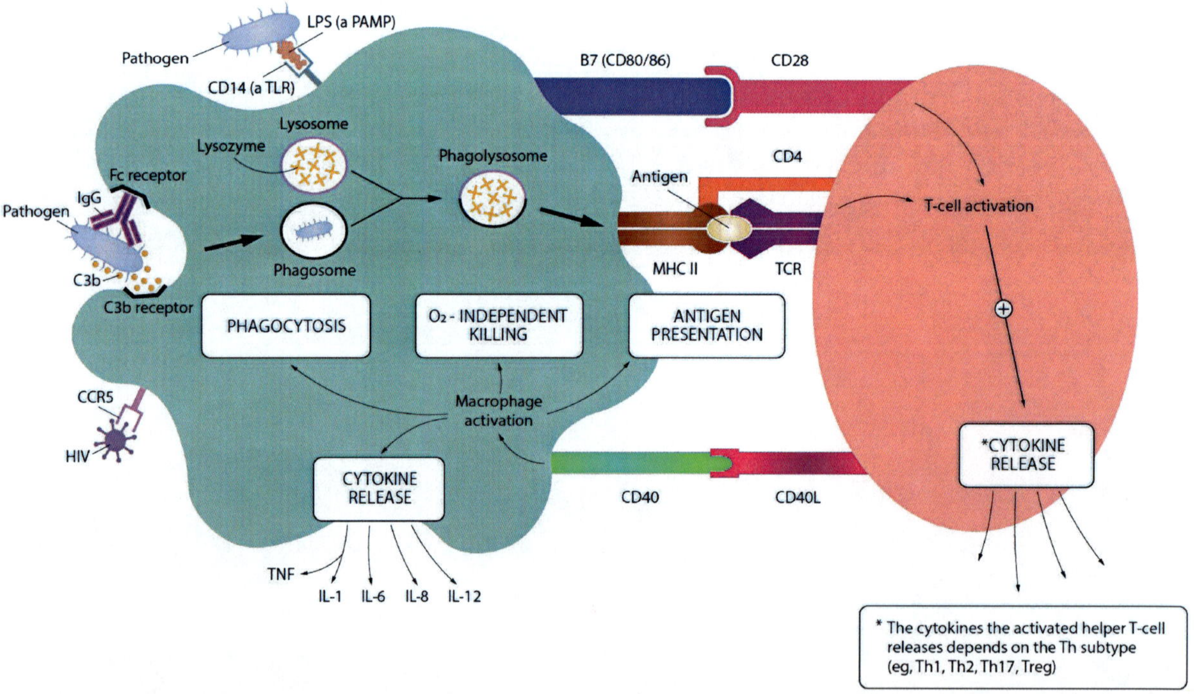

Figure 8.1.53 - Type IV hypersensitivity reaction (CD4+ T-cell mediated)

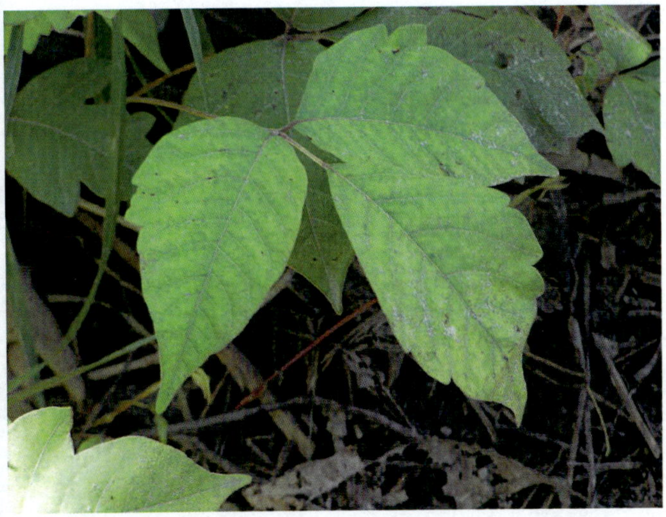

Photo Credit: Chris Light [CC BY-SA 4.0 (https://creativecommons.org/licenses/by-sa/4.0)]

II. Mechanism Mnemonic

A. Hypersensitivities = "ABCD"

1. Type I = anaphylactic and atopic
2. Type II = antibody mediated
3. Type III = immune complex
4. Type IV = delayed

REVIEW QUESTIONS ?

1. A 3-year-old boy is brought to the emergency department in anaphylactic shock after eating peanuts. Elevated serum concentrations of what substances can be used to support a diagnosis of anaphylaxis?

- **The correct answer is histamine and tryptase.**
- **This boy is in anaphylactic shock after eating peanuts.**
- **This is describing a type one hypersensitivity reaction.**
- **In a type one reaction, mast cells degranulate and release histamine along with tryptase.**
- **Both serum histamine and tryptase concentrations can be assessed to support a diagnosis of anaphylaxis because it indicates that widespread mast cell degranulation is occuring.**

Section XVI - Blood Transfusion Reactions

Type	Description	Timing	Clinical Presentation	Notes
Anaphylactic reaction	Reaction against plasma proteins in transfused blood; common in patients with selective IgA deficiency (complete mechanism unknown)	Within minutes to 2-3 hours	Fever, urticaria, hypotension, pruritus respiratory symptoms, shock (anaphylaxis)	Type I hypersensitivity reaction; avoid blood products with IgA
Acute hemolytic transfusion reaction	1. Intravascular hemolysis - host IgM and/or MAC induce hemolysis of donor RBCs 2. Extravascular hemolysis - host antibody binds to donor RBCs which leads to phagocytosis	Within 1 hour	Chills, fever, hypotension, hemoglobinuria, renal failure, tachycardia, jaundice (extravascular)	Type II hypersensitivity reaction
Febrile nonhemolytic transfusion reaction	1. Cytokines are produced and accumulate while blood products are stored 2. Host antibodies are directed against donor HLA and WBCs	Within 1-6 hours	Mild fever, flushing, headaches, chills, mild dyspnea	Reaction prevented by filtering white blood cells before transfusion (leukoreduction)
Transfusion-related acute lung injury (TRALI)	Acute lung injury that occurs during or after blood product administration; Donor anti-leukocyte antibodies against recipient pulmonary endothelial cells and PMNs	Within 6 hours	Noncardiogenic pulmonary edema and respiratory distress	Rare

Table 8.1.8 - Blood transfusion reactions

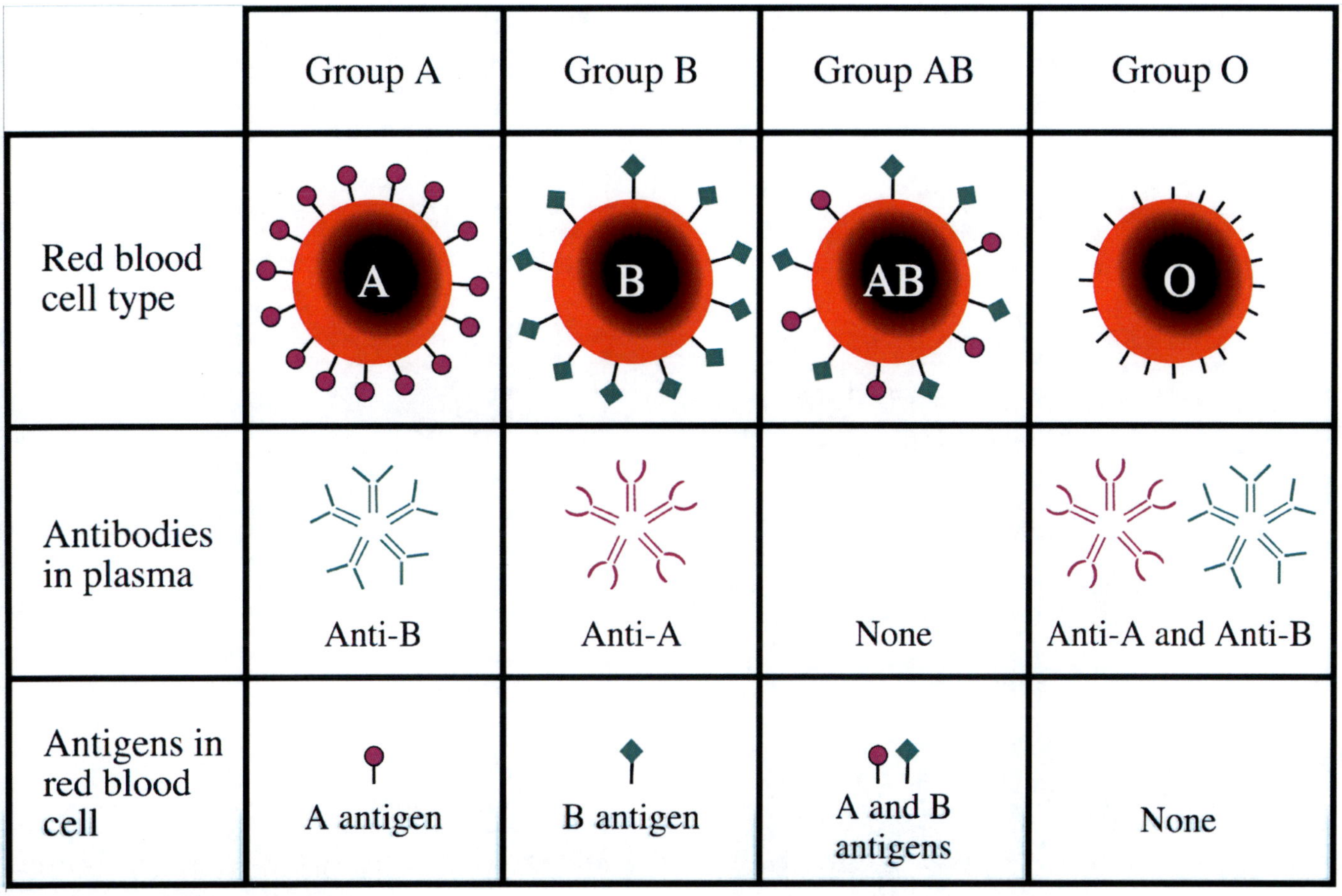

Photo Credit: InvictaHOG [Public Domain]

Figure 8.1.54 - Blood types

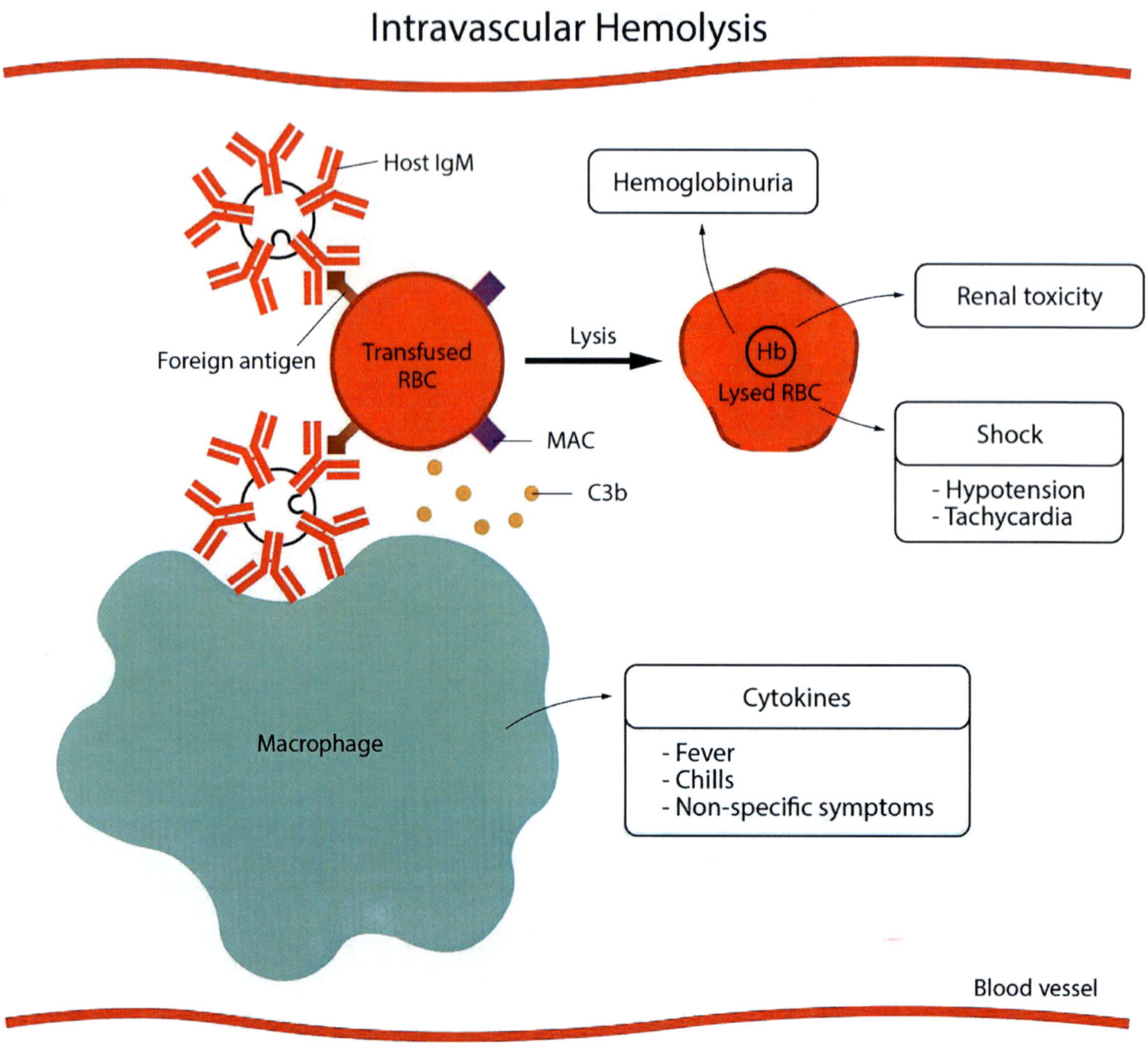

Figure 8.1.55 - Intravascular hemolysis

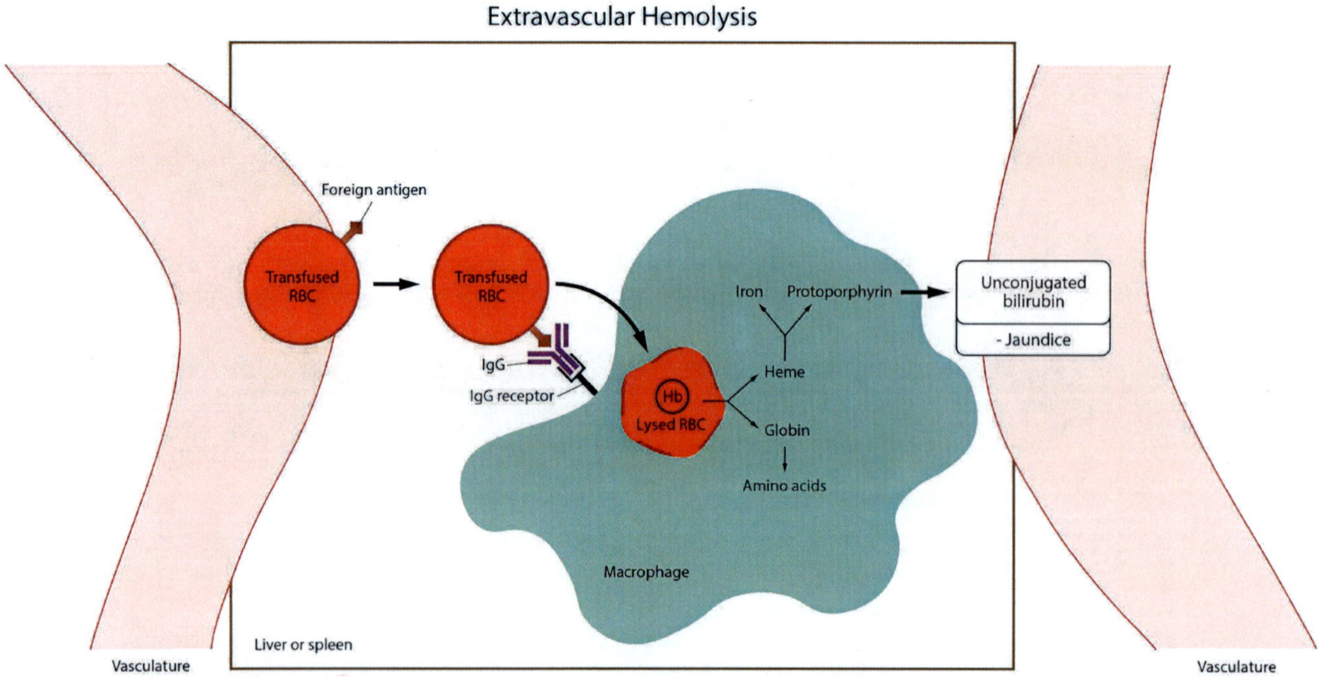

Figure 8.1.56 - Extravascular hemolysis

REVIEW QUESTIONS

?

1. A 57-year-old male undergoing an abdominal aortic aneurysm repair receives 2 liters of blood. Within 30 minutes the patient develops a temperature of 38.7°C (101.6°F) and his blood pressure drops to 80/40 mmHg. A direct Coombs test is positive. What type of transfusion reaction explains these findings?

- **Correct answer: acute hemolytic transfusion reaction**
- **This patient received 2 liters of blood and then developed a fever of 38.7°C and became hypotensive with a blood pressure of 80/40.**
- **Finally, he had a positive direct Coombs test.**
- **Recall that a positive direct Coombs test means that antibodies have attached directly to the surface of red blood cells.**
- **In other words, we can deduce that the reaction must have been caused by host antibodies that attached to donor red blood cells.**
- **This is describing an acute hemolytic transfusion reaction.**
- **From the table, we can see that an acute hemolytic transfusion reaction occurs when antibodies form against red blood cell antigens.**
- **So in the case of our patient he most likely received red blood cells that were incompatible with his blood type, resulting in intravascular hemolysis.**

Section XVII - Transplant Rejection

I. Transplant

A. Transplant:

1. Biological object transferred from one anatomical site to another (not limited to organs)

B. Graft:

1. Transplanted material

Type	Description	Example
Autograft	Transplantation from self to self	Skin graft of burn patient
Syngraft or isograft	Transplantation between identical twins	Kidney transplant between identical twins
Allograft	Transplantation between nonidentical individuals of the same species	Blood transfusion between two humans
Xenogeneic graft	Transplantation between two individuals of different species	Cardiac valves from pig to human

Table 8.1.9 - Graft types

II. Graft Success

A. Several markers must be evaluated to prevent graft rejection:

1. ABO blood group
2. HLA similarity between donor and recipient

B. Immunosuppressants

1. Prevent reaction between graft and donor
2. Host becomes immunocompromised

Type of Rejection	Description	Onset	Histology	Notes
Hyperacute	- Pre-existing host antibodies react to ABO and/or HLA antigens → complement activation	- Minutes to hours	- Thrombosis of graft vessels - Ischemia - Necrosis	- Type II hypersensitivity reaction - Graft must be removed
Acute	- Cellular: CD4+ and CD8+ T-cells are activated in response to graft - Humoral: B-cells differentiate into plasma cells and produce antibodies against graft (similar to hyperacute but takes longer)	- Weeks to months	- Dense lymphocytic infiltrate - Vasculitis of graft vessels	- Type II (humoral) and IV (cellular) hypersensitivity reactions - Can be prevented or reversed with immunosuppressants
Chronic	- Cellular and humoral response - CD4+ T-cells react to recipient APCs presenting donor peptides, including allogeneic APCs - Cytokines from T-cells induce histological changes	- Months to years	- Vascular smooth muscle proliferation - Luminal narrowing - Arteriosclerosis - Parenchymal atrophy - Interstitial fibrosis	- Type II (humoral) and IV (cellular) hypersensitivity reactions

Table 8.1.10 - Types of Transplant Rejection

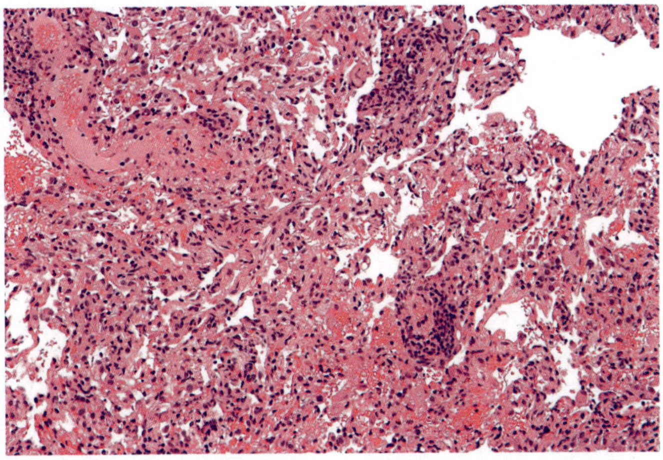

Photo Credit: Nephron [CC BY-SA 3.0 (https://creativecommons.org/licenses/by-sa/3.0)]

C. Acute rejection reaction (dense lymphocytic infiltrate)

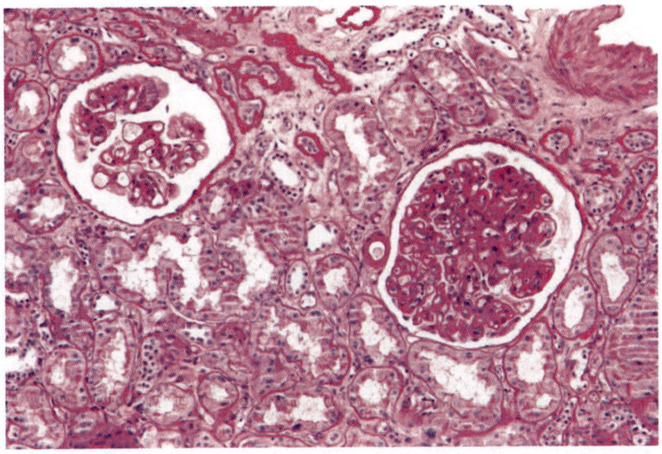

Photo Credit: Nephron [CC BY-SA 3.0 (https://creativecommons.org/licenses/by-sa/3.0)]

D. Chronic rejection reaction (narrowing of the blood vessels and interstitial fibrosis)

III. Graft vs. Host Disease

A. Rejection initiated by donor T-cells in an immunosuppressed host

1. Severe organ dysfunction
2. Type IV hypersensitivity reaction

B. Jaundice, rash, diarrhea, hepatosplenomegaly

C. Common in bone marrow transplant patients

D. May be beneficial in bone marrow transplant (grafted T-cells kill residual host cancer cells)

E. Prevent by irradiating blood products prior to transfusion

REVIEW QUESTIONS

1. An 18-year-old male with a history of polycystic kidney disease receives a kidney transplant. Three weeks later he develops a fever and tenderness at the costovertebral angle. Laboratory work reveals a rise in creatinine. A biopsy of this patient's transplanted kidney will most likely reveal what histological changes?

- **The answer to the question is a dense lymphocytic infiltrate.**
- **This patient has had problems three weeks after receiving a kidney transplant.**
- **Remember, the timing is the most important part of this question because it tells you what type of rejection is going on.**
- **In this case, it must be an acute rejection.**
- **Hyperacute rejection occurs within minutes to hours, acute rejection occurs within weeks to months, and chronic rejection occurs within months to years.**
- **The timing means that this patient must have an acute rejection which is characterized by a dense lymphocytic infiltrate.**
- **Again, this just means that there will be a lot of lymphocytes seen on histology - mostly T lymphocytes.**

IMMUNODEFICIENCIES

Section I - Bruton Agammaglobulinemia

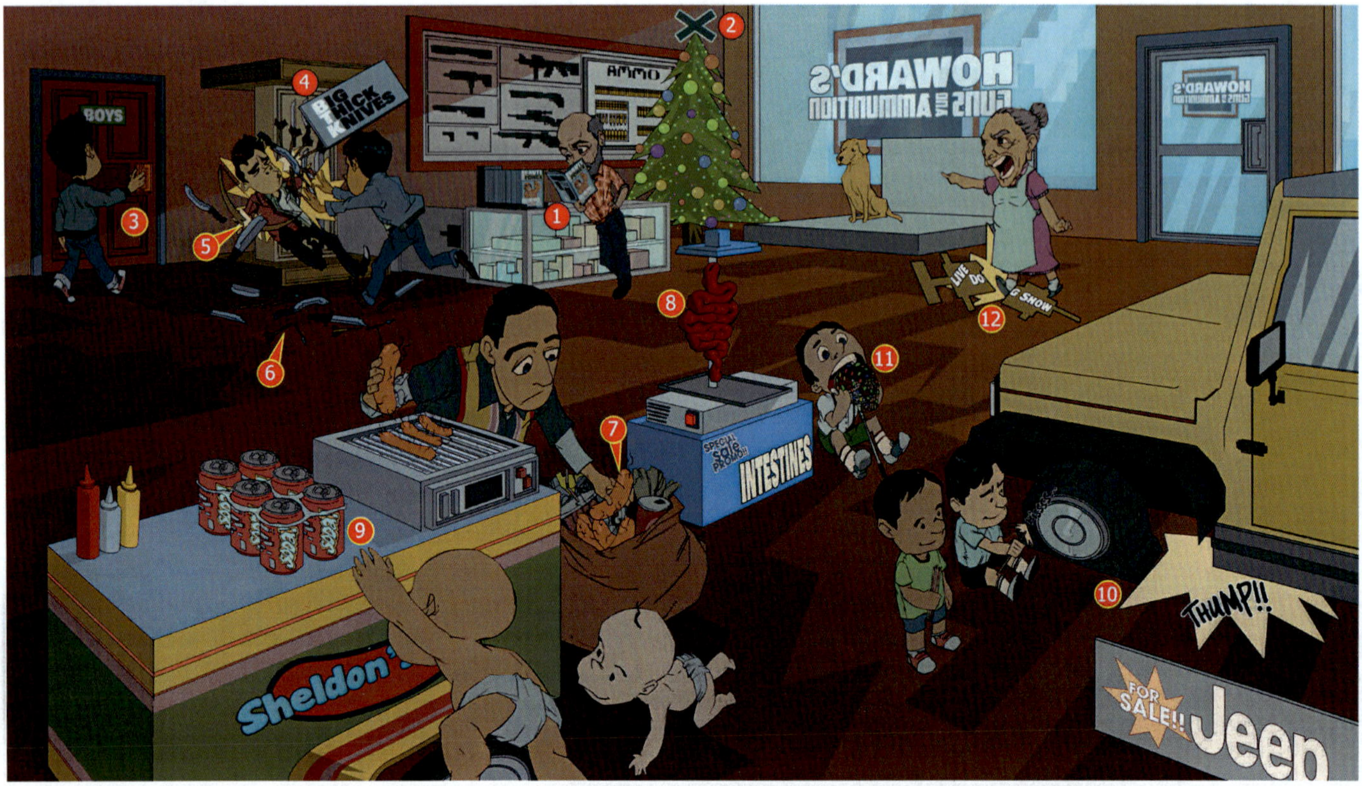

1. ______________________
2. ______________________
3. ______________________
4. ______________________
5. ______________________
6. ______________________
7. ______________________
8. ______________________
9. ______________________
10. ______________________
11. ______________________
12. ______________________

Section II - Selective IgA Deficiency

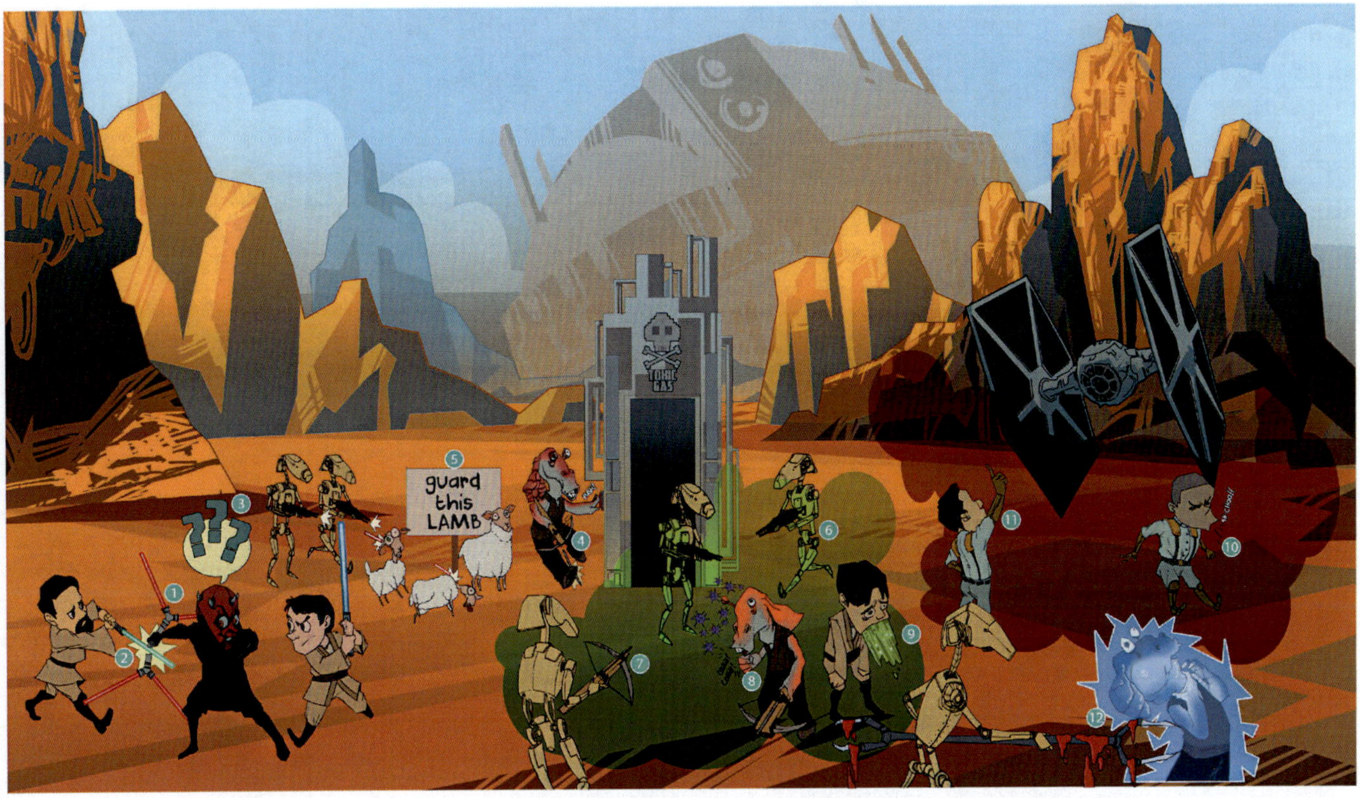

1. ______________________
2. ______________________
3. ______________________
4. ______________________
5. ______________________
6. ______________________
7. ______________________
8. ______________________
9. ______________________
10. ______________________
11. ______________________
12. ______________________

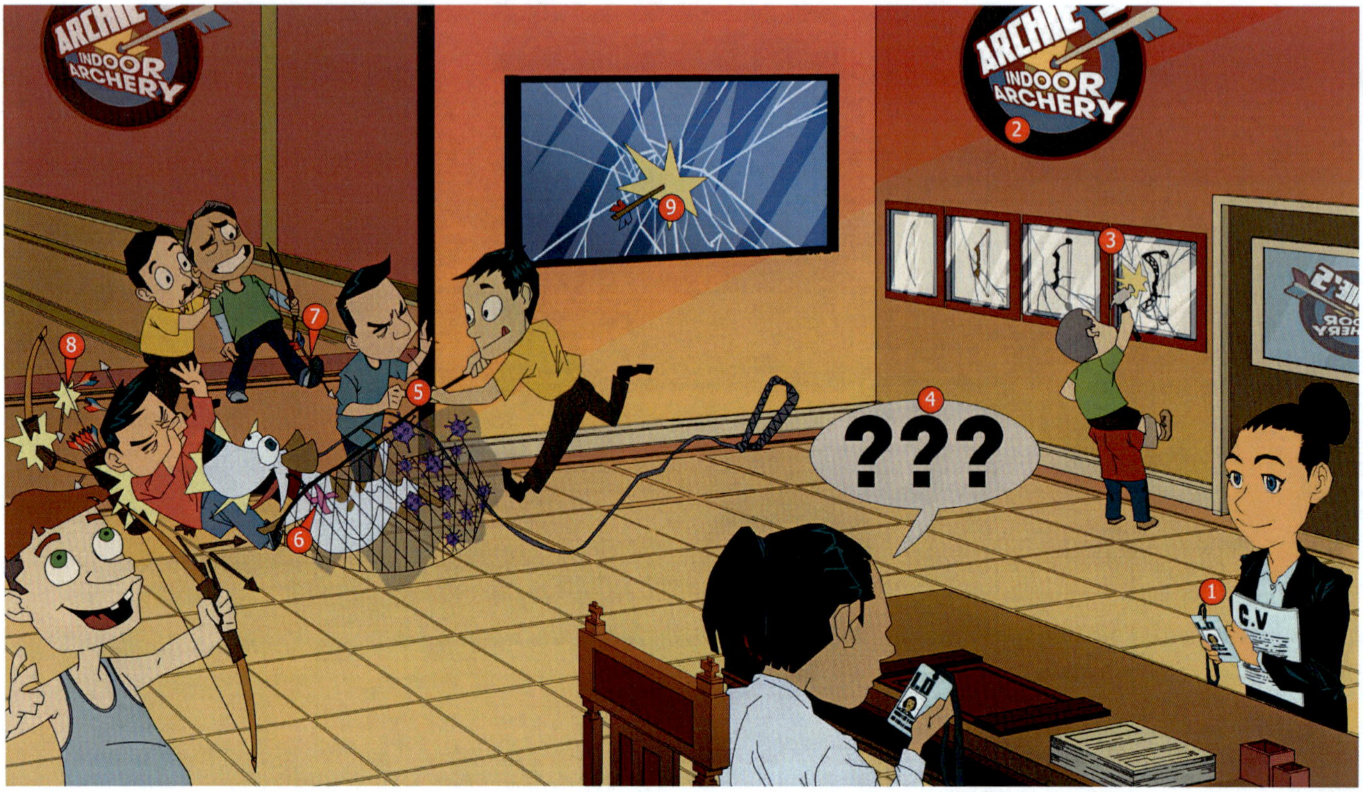

1. ______________________
2. ______________________
3. ______________________
4. ______________________
5. ______________________
6. ______________________
7. ______________________
8. ______________________
9. ______________________

Section IV - Thymic Aplasia

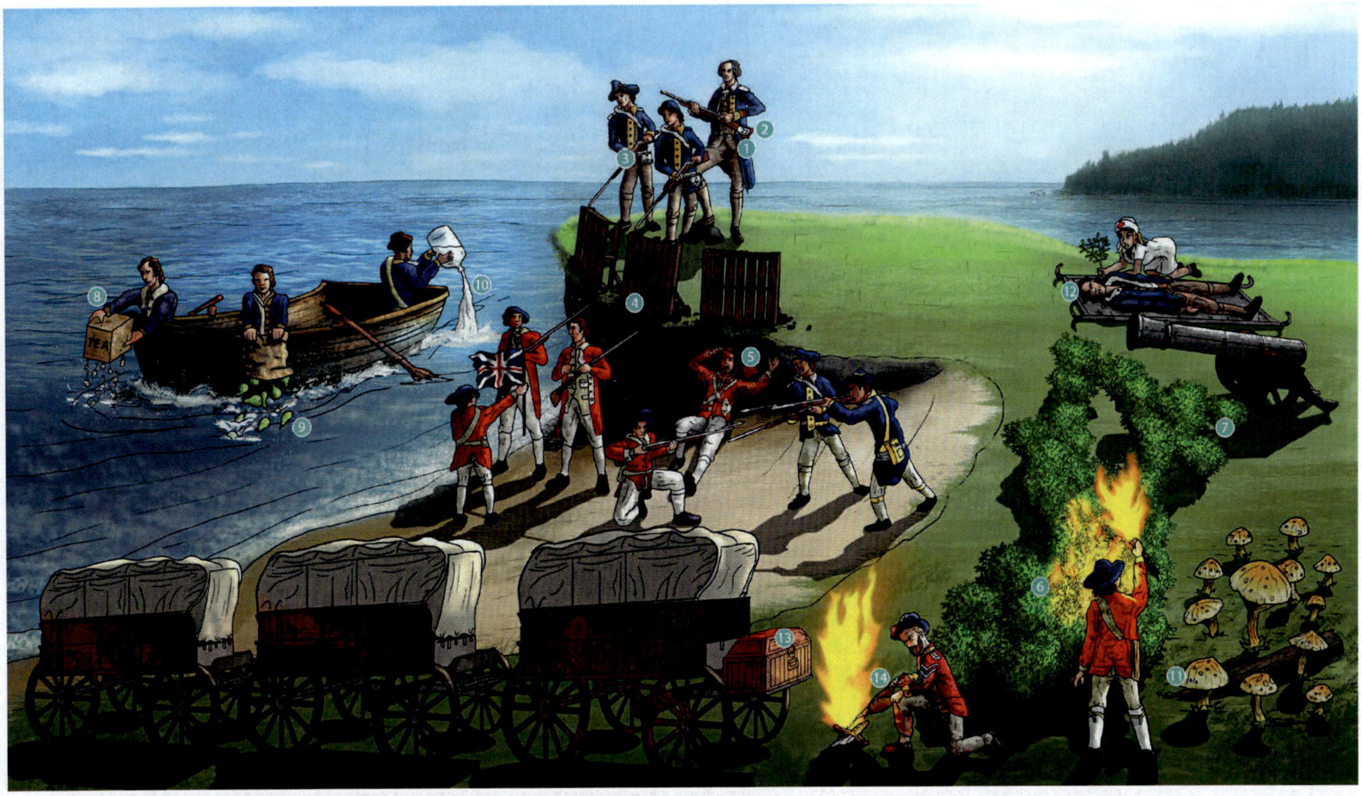

1. ______________________
2. ______________________
3. ______________________
4. ______________________
5. ______________________
6. ______________________
7. ______________________
8. ______________________
9. ______________________
10. ______________________
11. ______________________
12. ______________________
13. ______________________
14. ______________________

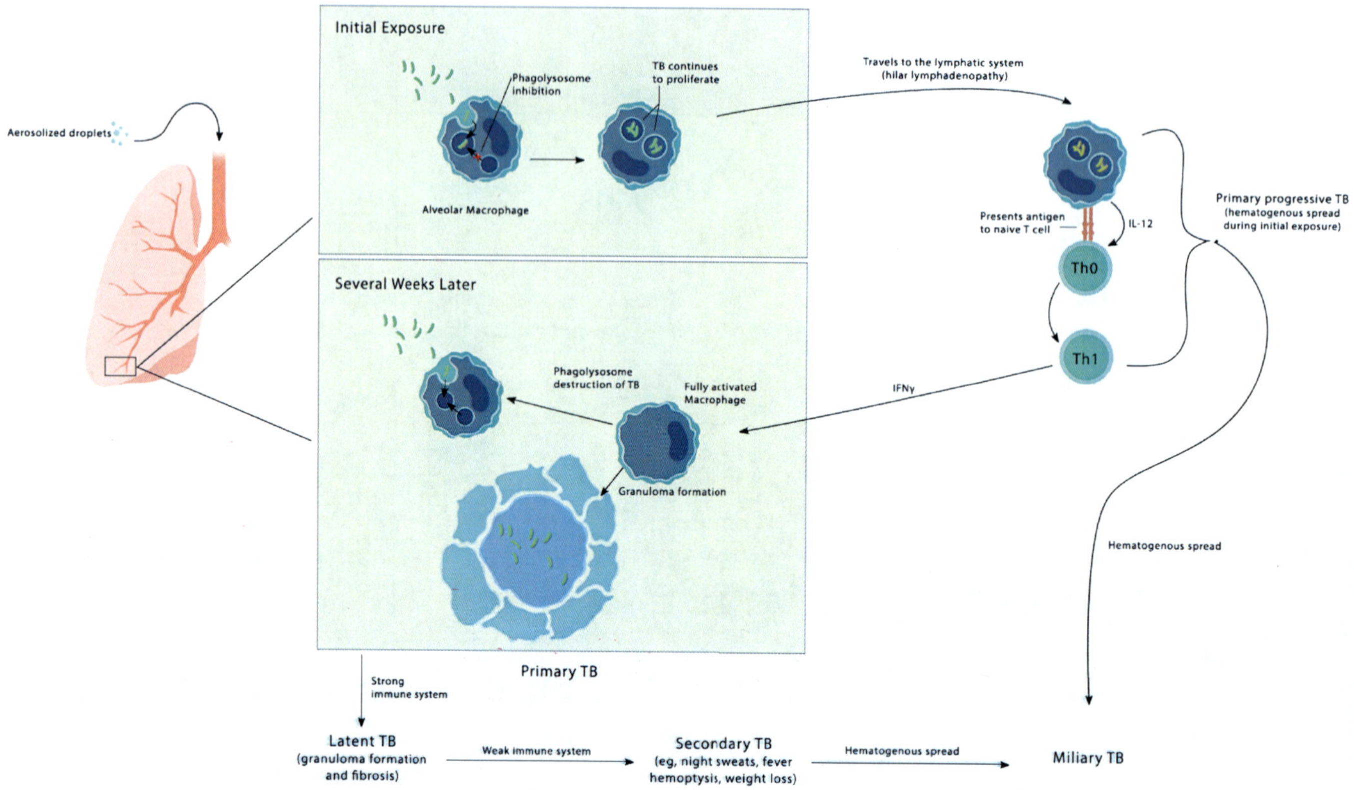

Figure 8.2.1 - Pathophysiology of *Mycobacterium tuberculosis*

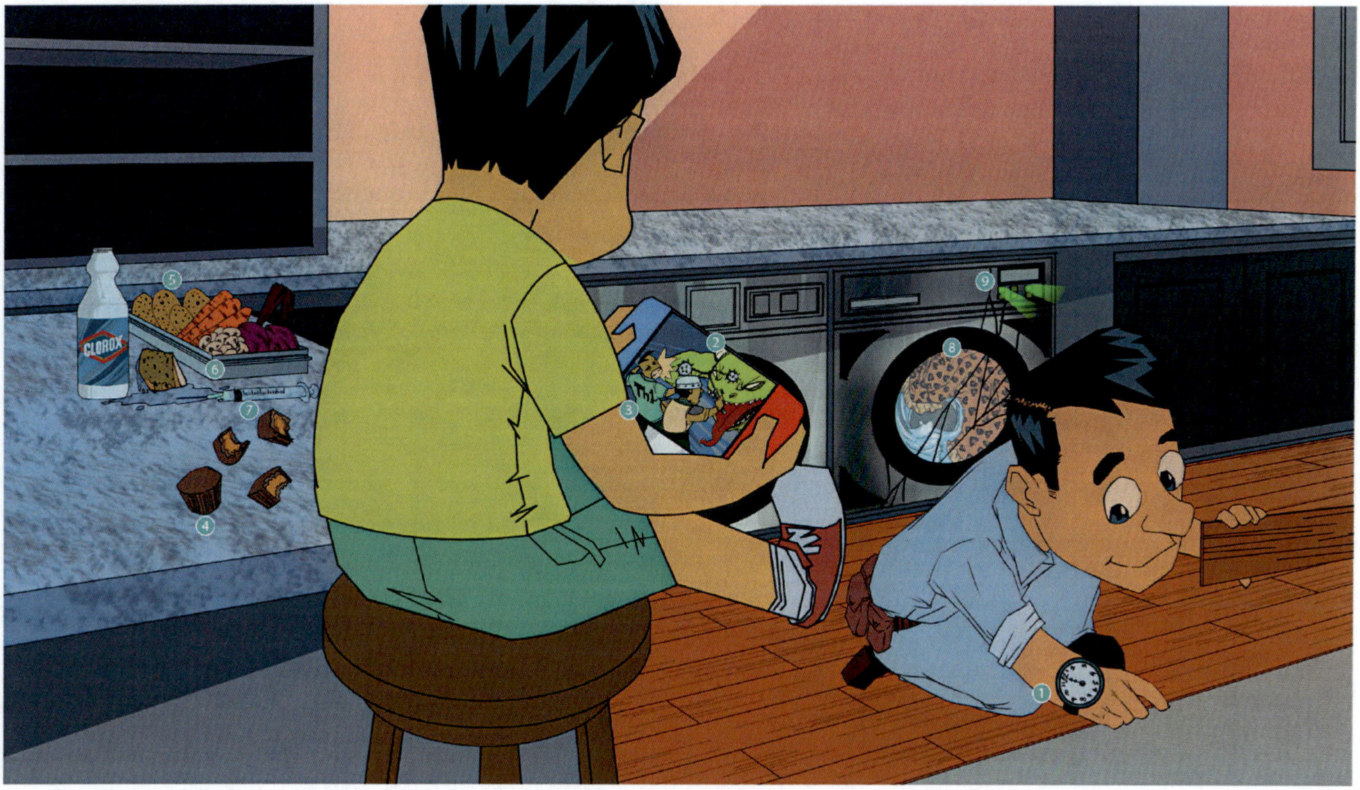

1. ____________________
2. ____________________
3. ____________________
4. ____________________
5. ____________________
6. ____________________
7. ____________________
8. ____________________
9. ____________________

Section VI - Job Syndrome

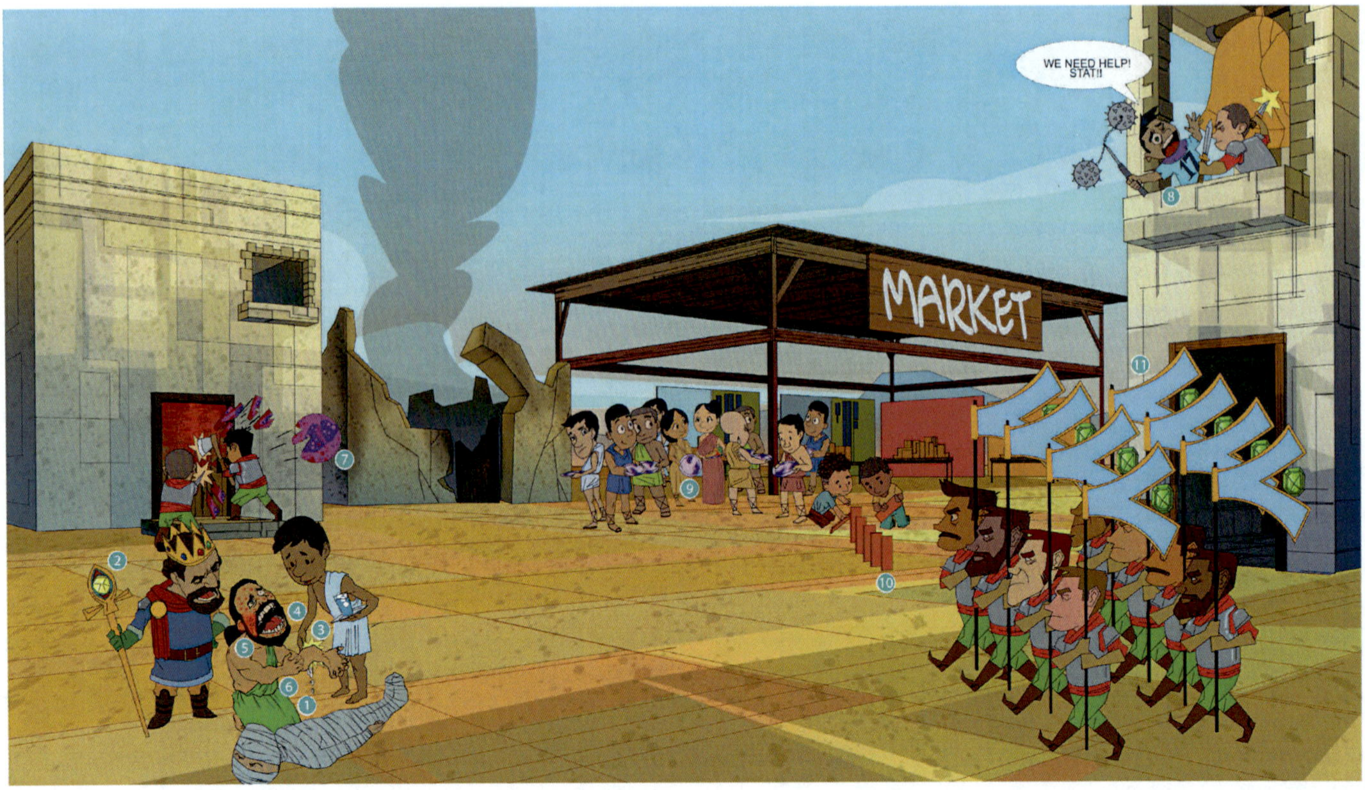

1. ______________________
2. ______________________
3. ______________________
4. ______________________
5. ______________________
6. ______________________
7. ______________________
8. ______________________
9. ______________________
10. ______________________
11. ______________________

Section VII - Chronic mucocutaneous candidiasis

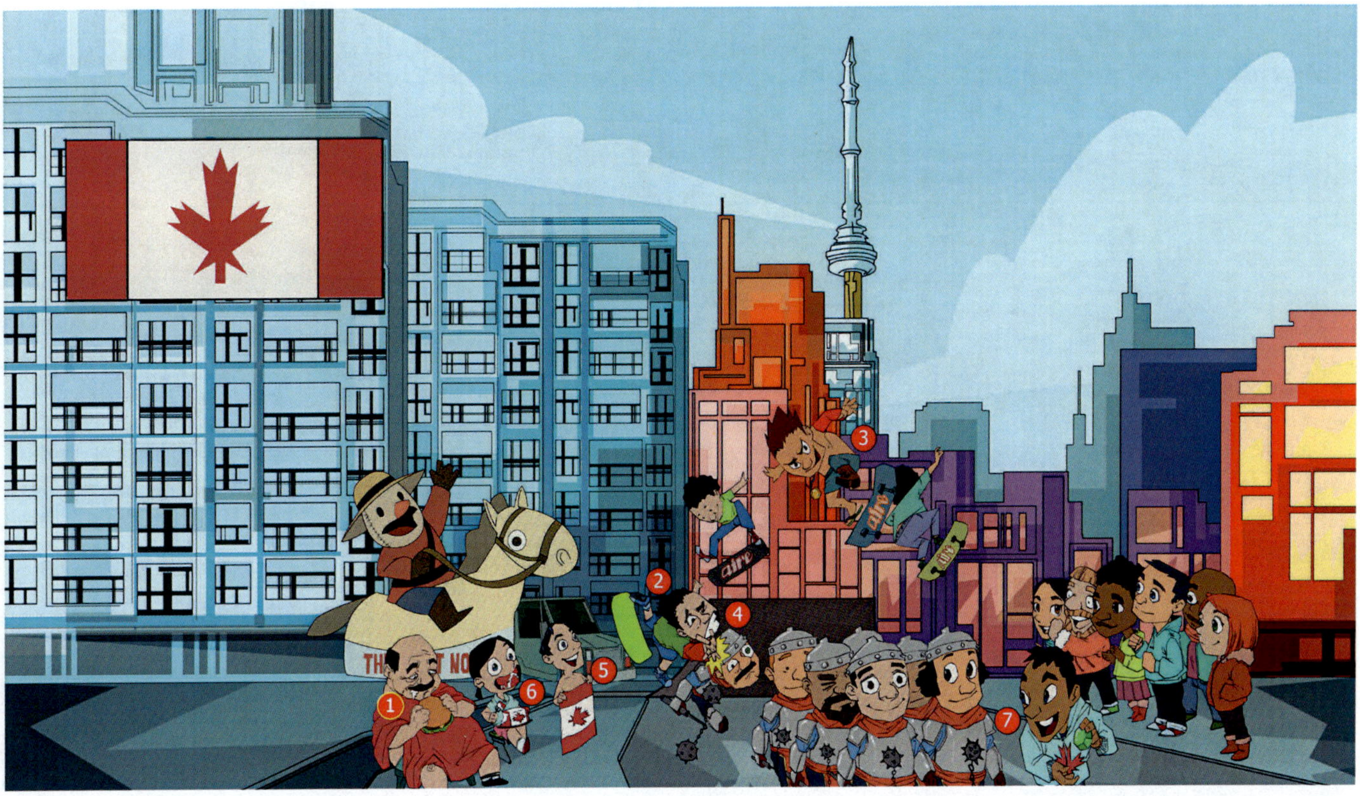

1. ____________________

2. ____________________

3. ____________________

4. ____________________

5. ____________________

6. ____________________

7. ____________________

Section VIII - Severe combined immunodeficiency (SCID)

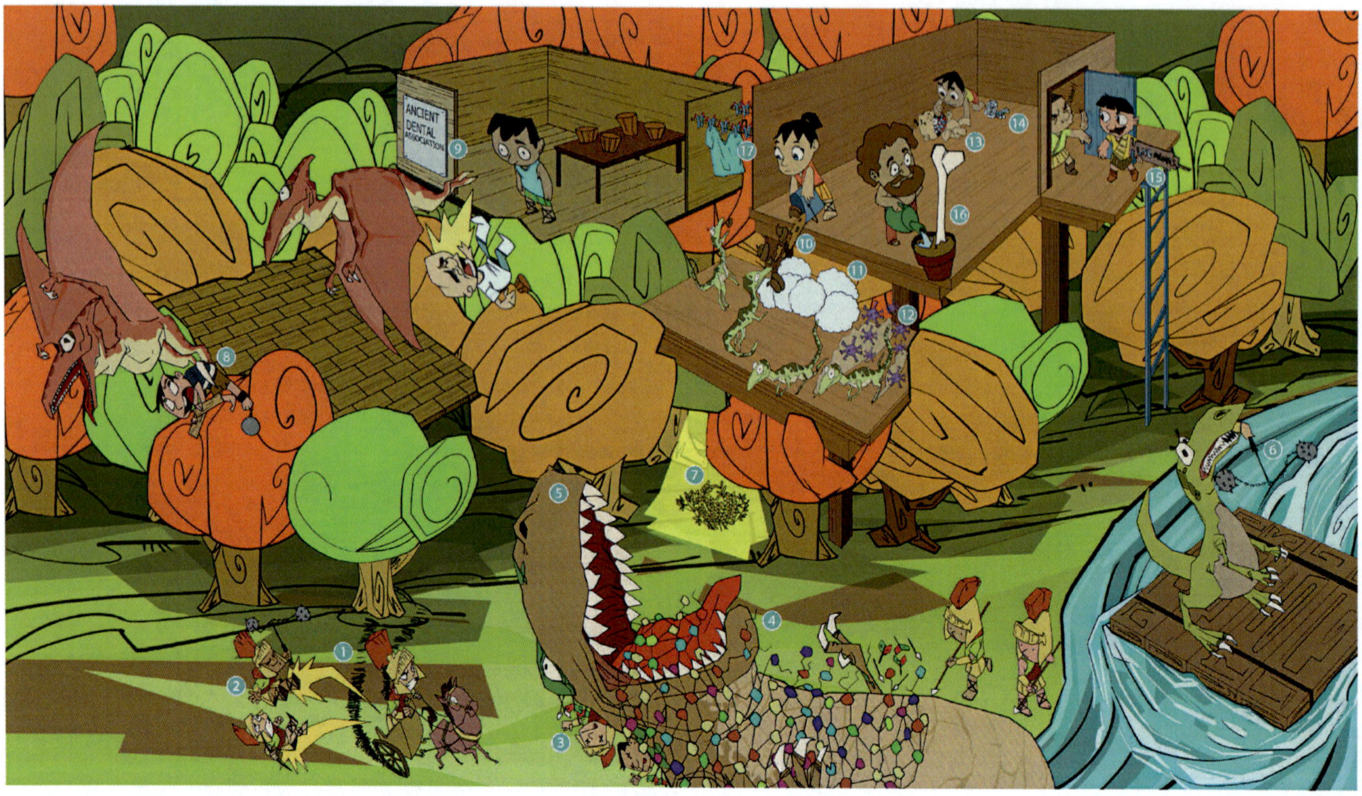

1. ______________________________
2. ______________________________
3. ______________________________
4. ______________________________
5. ______________________________
6. ______________________________
7. ______________________________
8. ______________________________
9. ______________________________
10. ______________________________
11. ______________________________
12. ______________________________
13. ______________________________
14. ______________________________
15. ______________________________
16. ______________________________
17. ______________________________

Section IX - Ataxia-telangiectasia

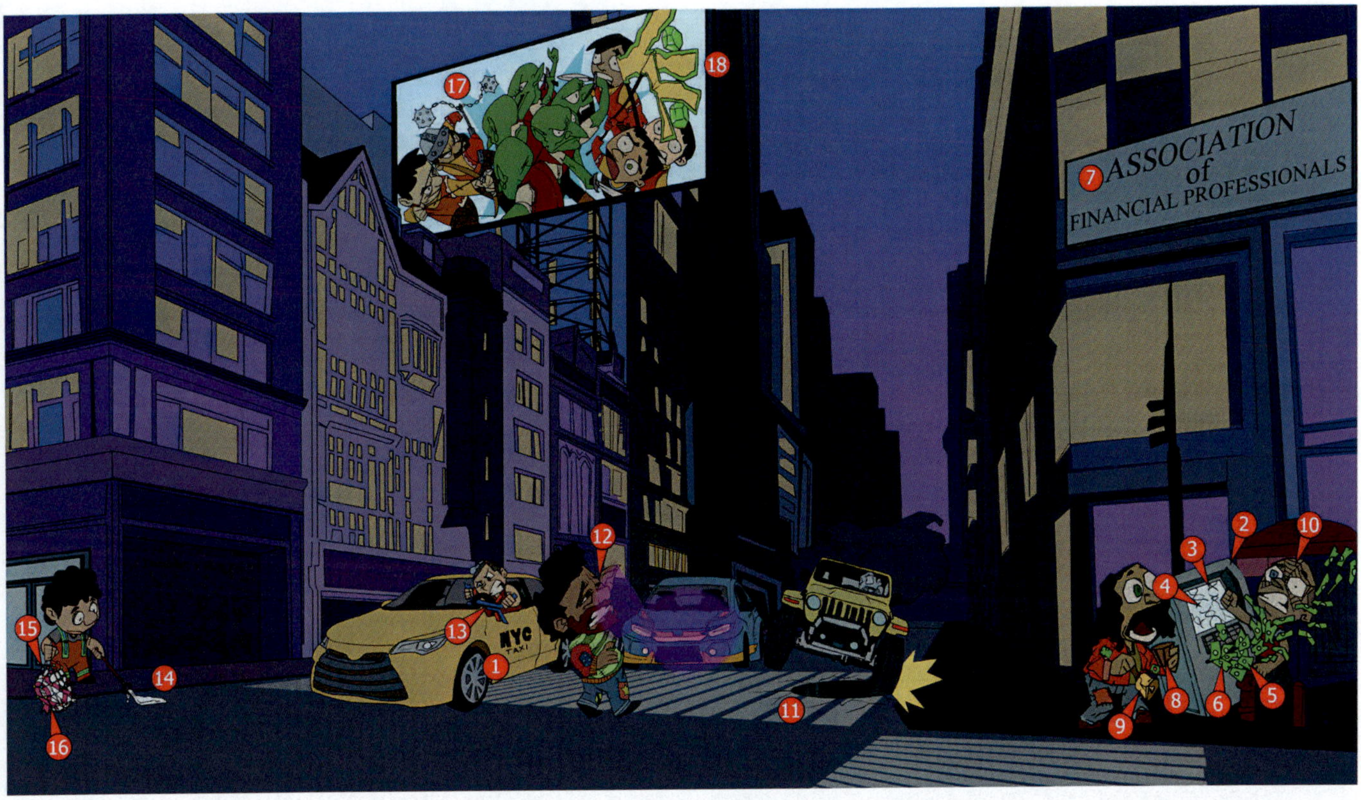

1. ______________________________
2. ______________________________
3. ______________________________
4. ______________________________
5. ______________________________
6. ______________________________
7. ______________________________
8. ______________________________
9. ______________________________
10. ______________________________
11. ______________________________
12. ______________________________
13. ______________________________
14. ______________________________
15. ______________________________
16. ______________________________
17. ______________________________
18. ______________________________

Section X - Hyper-IgM syndrome

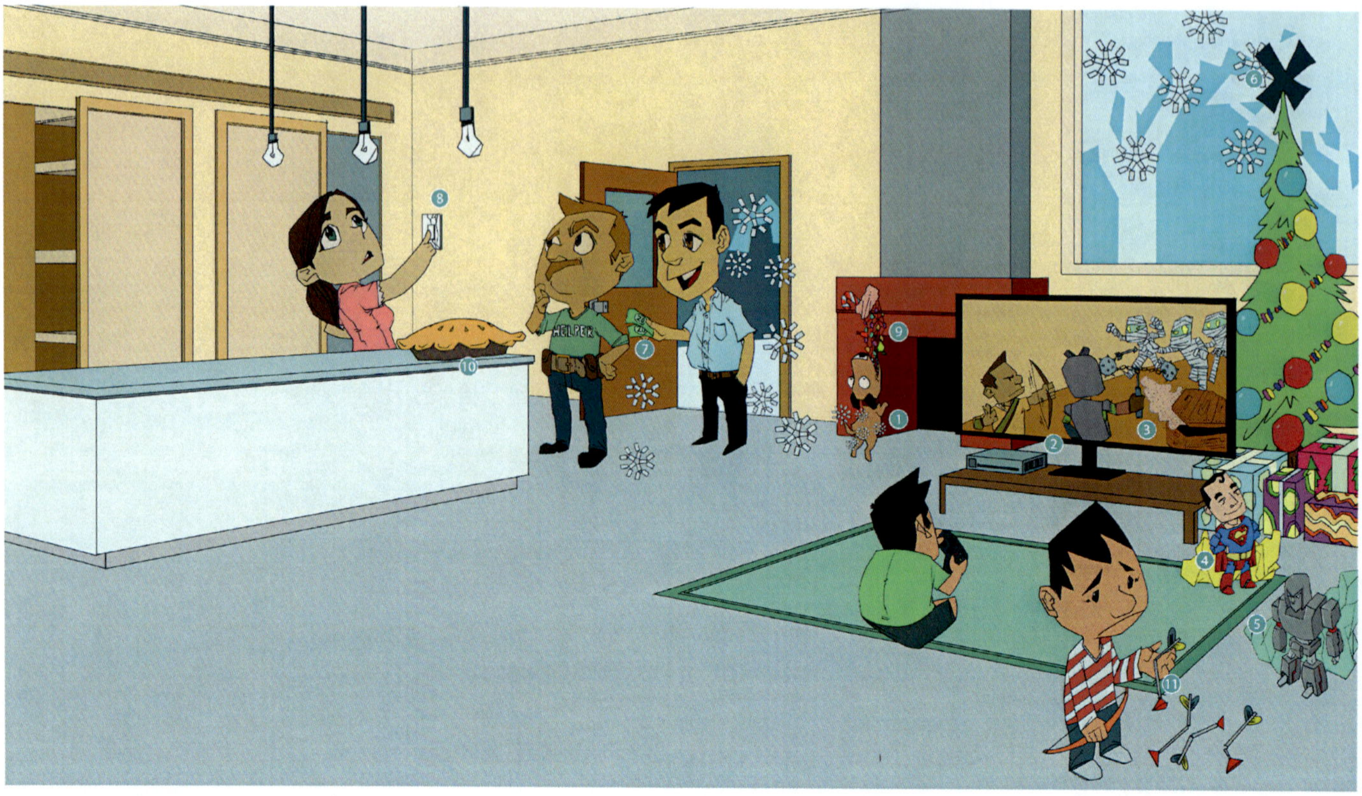

1. ____________________
2. ____________________
3. ____________________
4. ____________________
5. ____________________
6. ____________________
7. ____________________
8. ____________________
9. ____________________
10. ____________________
11. ____________________

Section XI - Wiskott-Aldrich Syndrome

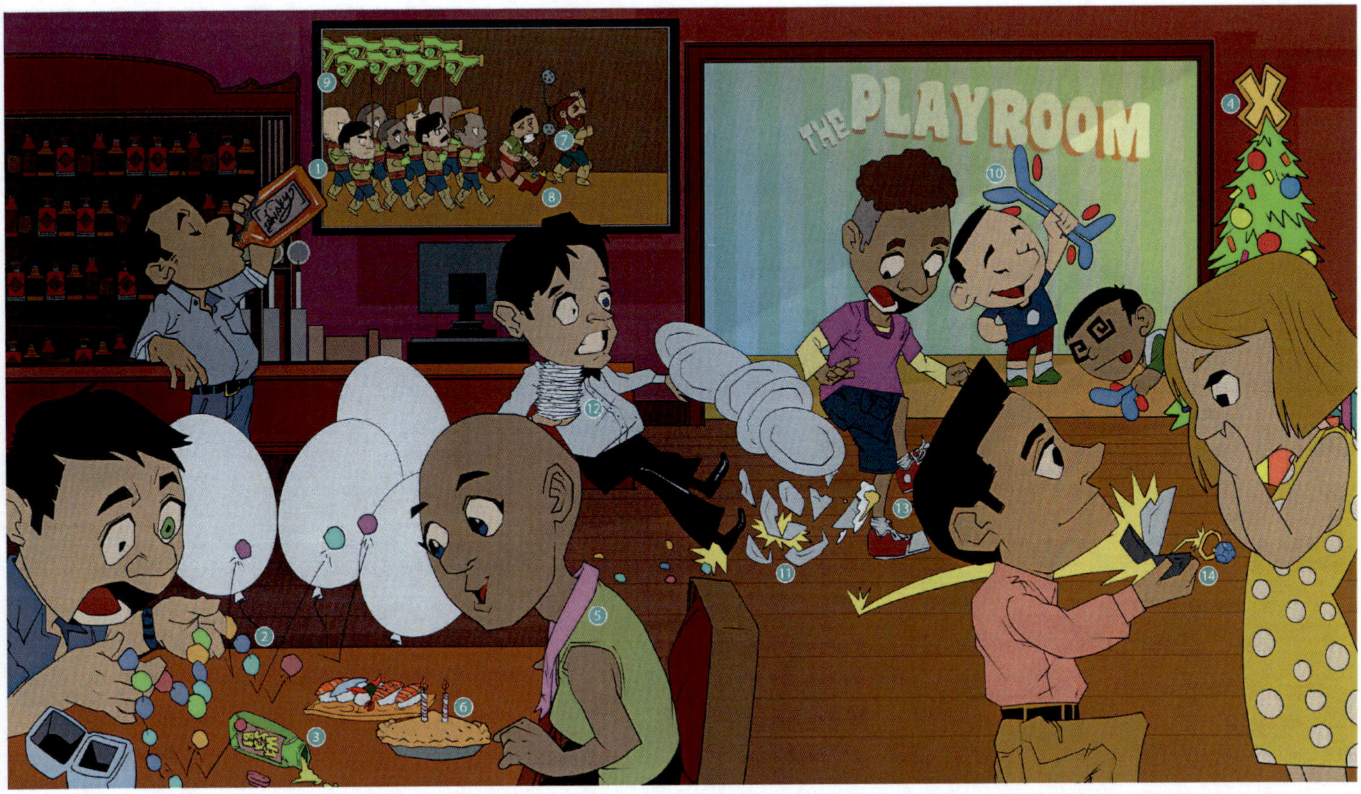

1. ______________________
2. ______________________
3. ______________________
4. ______________________
5. ______________________
6. ______________________
7. ______________________
8. ______________________
9. ______________________
10. ______________________
11. ______________________
12. ______________________
13. ______________________
14. ______________________

Section XII - Leukocyte Adhesion Deficiency

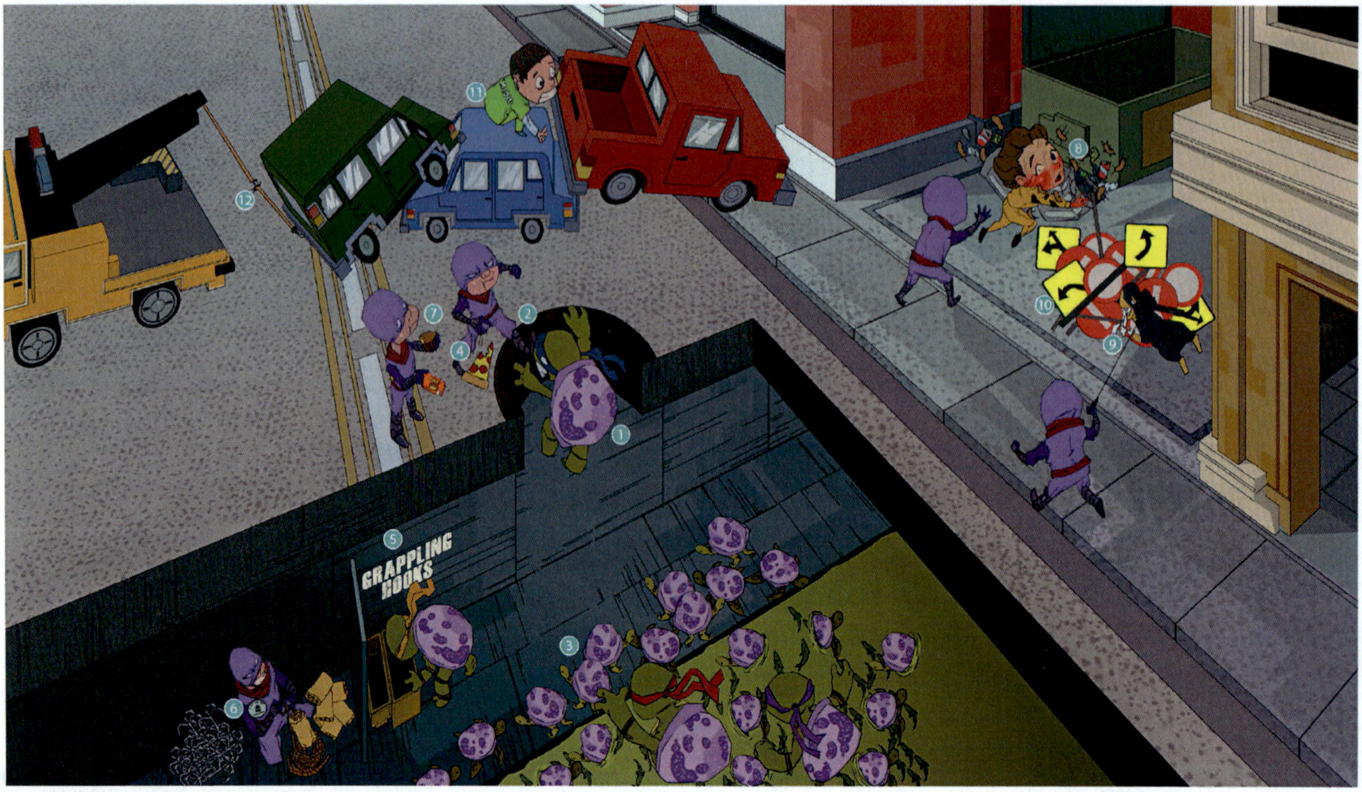

1. ______________________
2. ______________________
3. ______________________
4. ______________________
5. ______________________
6. ______________________
7. ______________________
8. ______________________
9. ______________________
10. ______________________
11. ______________________
12. ______________________

Section XIII - Chediak-Higashi syndrome

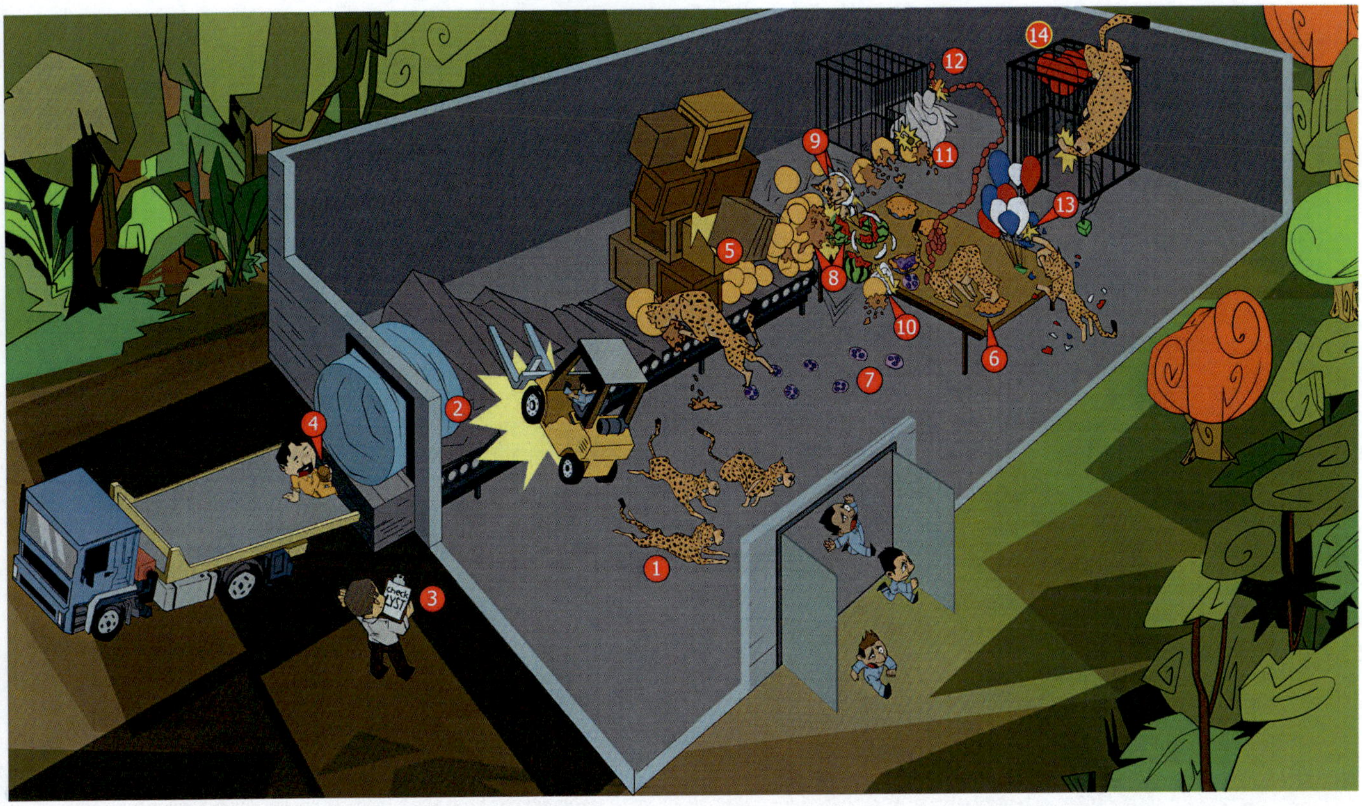

1. ______________________
2. ______________________
3. ______________________
4. ______________________
5. ______________________
6. ______________________
7. ______________________
8. ______________________
9. ______________________
10. ______________________
11. ______________________
12. ______________________
13. ______________________
14. ______________________

Section XIV - Chronic Granulomatous Disease

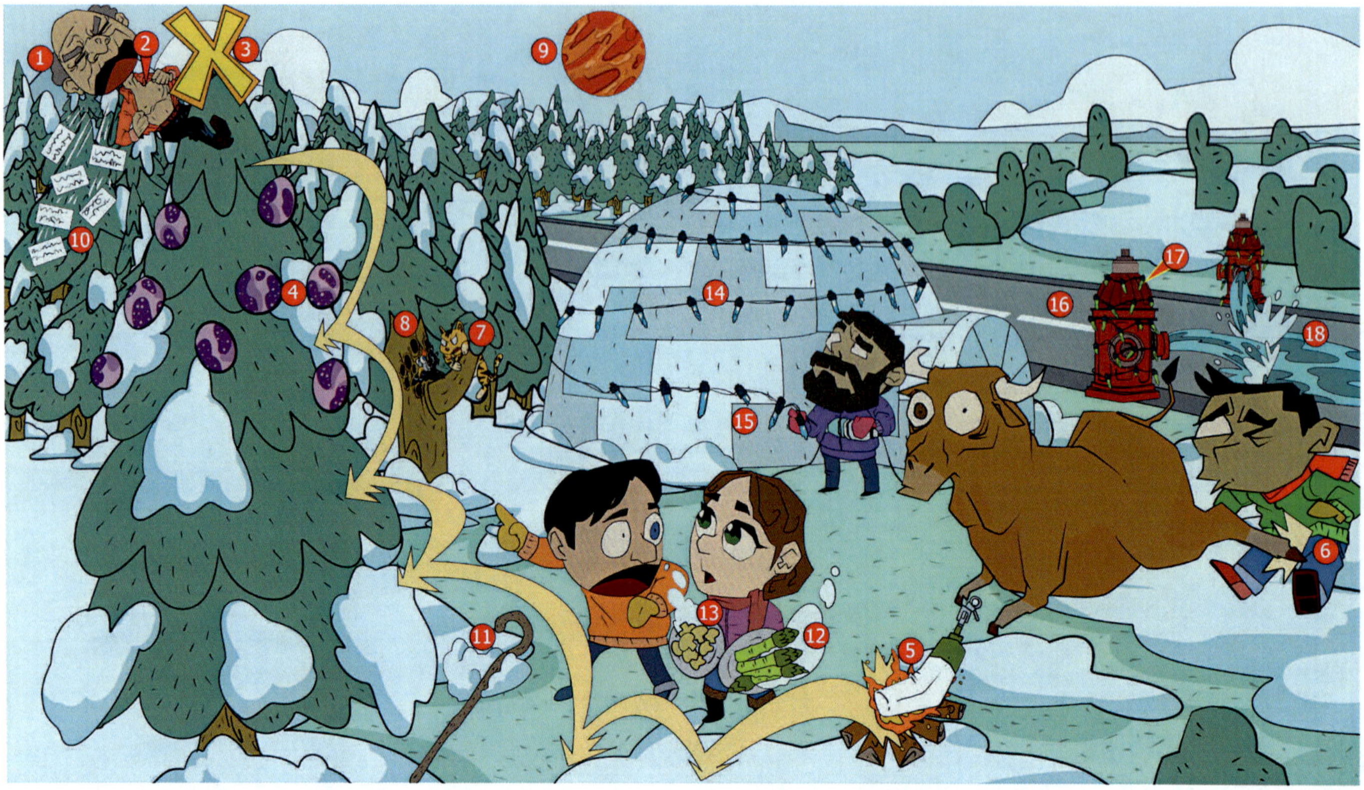

1. ______________________
2. ______________________
3. ______________________
4. ______________________
5. ______________________
6. ______________________
7. ______________________
8. ______________________
9. ______________________
10. ______________________
11. ______________________
12. ______________________
13. ______________________
14. ______________________
15. ______________________
16. ______________________
17. ______________________
18. ______________________

Made in United States
North Haven, CT
04 November 2026

21736872R00049